Cardiovascular and Respiratory Physiology in the Fetus and Neonate

Physiologie Cardiovasculaire et Respiratoire du Fœtus et du Nouveau-Né

Colloques INSERM
ISSN 0768-3154

Other *Colloques* published by John Libbey Eurotext and INSERM

133 Cardiovascular and Respiratory Physiology in the Fetus and Neonate. Scientific Committee: P. Karlberg, A. Minkowski, W. Oh & L. Stern; Managing Editor: M. Monset-Couchard
ISBN 0 98196 086 6 (INSERM ISBN 2 85598 282 0)

134 Porphyrins and Porphyrias. Edited by Y. Nordmann
ISBN 0 86196 087 4 (INSERM ISBN 2 85598 281 2)

137 Neo-Adjuvant Chemotherapy. Edited by Claude Jacquillat, Marise Weil & David Khayat
ISBN 0 86196 077 7 (INSERM ISBN 2 85598 283 9)

139 Hormones and Cell Regulation. Edited by Jacques Nunez & Jacques E. Dumont
ISBN 0 86196 084 X (INSERM ISBN 2 85598 284 7)

Cardiovascular and Respiratory Physiology in the Fetus and Neonate

Physiologie Cardiovasculaire et Respiratoire du Fœtus et du Nouveau-Né

Proceedings of the international conference held in Paris (France)
20-29 January 1985

Sponsored by the Institut National de la Santé et de la Recherche Médicale

Scientific Committee
P. Karlberg
A. Minkowski
W. Oh
L. Stern

Managing Editor
M. Monset-Couchard

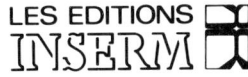

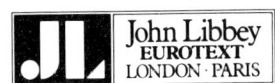

British Library Cataloguing in Publication Data
Cardiovascular and respiratory physiology in the fetus and
   neonate: proceedings of the John Lind Memorial Conference,
   Paris, 1985.—(Les colloques de l'INSERM Volume 133)
   1. Fetus—Physiology   2. Infants (Newborn)—Physiology
   3. Cardiovascular system   4. Fetal heart
   5. Fetus—Respiration and cry   6. Respiratory organs
   I. Titla   II. Couchard, M.   III. Series
   612'.1   RG618

ISBN 0-86196-086-6
ISSN 0768-3154

First published in 1986 by

John Libbey & Company Ltd
80/84 Bondway, London SW8 1SF, England. (01) 582 5266
John Libbey Eurotext Ltd
6 rue Blanche, 92120 Montrouge, France. (1) 47 35 85 52
ISBN 0 86196 086 6

Institut National de la Santé et de la Recherche Médicale
101 rue de Tolbiac, 75654 Paris Cedex 13, France. (1) 45 84 14 41
ISBN 2 85598 282 0

ISSN 0768-3154

© 1986 Colloques INSERM/John Libbey Eurotext Ltd
All rights reserved
Unauthorised duplication contravenes applicable laws

Typeset by Gwynnes, Hurstpierpoint, Sussex
Printed in Great Britain by
Whitstable Litho Ltd., Whitstable, Kent

Opening Remarks

To celebrate a great scientist, and an exceptional human being, constitutes, in our era of 'realpolitik' and materialism an unusual event.

To be able, on such an occasion, to organize a conference on a high academic level, accompanied by cultural events, is a new avenue in the field of meetings on advanced medicine. John Lind deserved this type of meeting.

Almost everybody was John Lind's either pupil or friend. Everybody was deeply concerned. The Americans, Scandinavians, and French were continuously enveloped in the 'spirit of medical science'. Fetal circulation, neonatal lung physiology, baroque instruments and chamber music, 'Space, form, and illusion' (by Jack Metcoff) seemed to be on an equally high level.

The location, the XVIIth century convent of Port-Royal, made it possible to have with us the image of Blaise Pascal who, in those old premises, elaborated the first theory of probabilities and designed one of the first calculators.

During those three days, John Lind's spirit was with us. We thank him for having been able, by his life, spirit, and his work, to have given us the opportunity to be together on earth and in heaven.

Paris, 29–30 January 1985

P. Karlberg
A. Minkowski
W. Oh
L. Stern

Acknowledgements

We are grateful to INSERM which sponsored this conference and has permitted the publication of this volume.

M. Monset-Couchard, M.D., INSERM Chargée de Recherches, was responsible for editing this book. Her usual skillfulness and conscience goes along with the whole idea of the Conference. She devoted herself to the work that she accomplished with full dedication.

We are grateful to G. Vicente, electronics Engineer at INSERM Unité 29 who was in charge of recording the sessions.

Contents
Sommaire

5 Opening remarks
Note préliminaire

6 Acknowledgements
Remerciements

11 John Lind 1909–1983

THE JOHN LIND MEMORIAL LECTURE
CONFERENCE D'OUVERTURE EN HOMMAGE A JOHN LIND

15 **A.M. Rudolph**
Venous return and cardiac output in the perinatal period
Le retour veineux et le débit cardiaque pendant la période périnatale

FETAL AND NEONATAL CIRCULATION
CIRCULATION FOETALE ET NEONATALE

33 **R.A. Arcilla**
Role of intracardiac streaming upon early cardiac development
Rôle des courants sanguins intracardiaques dans le développement cardiaque précoce

47 **D.M. Friedman**
Fetal echocardiography and Doppler blood flow studies
Echocardiographie foetale: examen du débit sanguin foetal par ultrasonographie Doppler

55 **S.Z. Walsh**
Fetal–neonatal circulation revisited
Revue d'ensemble de la circulation foetale et néonatale

67 **K.G. Rosén, K.R. Greene, K.-H. Hökegård, K. Karlsson, H. Lilja, K. Lindecratz and I. Kjellmer**
ST waveform analysis of the fetal ECG—a potent method for fetal surveillance? A presentation of experimental and clinical data
L'analyse des ondes ST de l'ECG foetal est-elle une méthode efficace de surveillance du foetus? Présentation de données expérimentales et cliniques

83 **W. Oh**
Neonatal polycythaemia and hyperviscosity: the pathophysiological role of placental transfusion
Polycythémie et hyperviscosité néonatales: rôle pathophysiologique de la transfusion placentaire

NEONATAL PERIPHERAL CIRCULATION
CIRCULATION PERIPHERIQUE CHEZ LE NOUVEAU-NE

95 **B. Friis-Hansen**
Cerebral blood flow in the newborn infant
Débit sanguin cérébral chez le nouveau-né

109 **B.P.W. Lundell, H. Sundell, D.P. Lindstrom and M.T. Stahlman**
An animal model for measurements of intracranial blood flow velocities
Modèle expérimental de mesure des vélocités du courant sanguin intracranien chez l'animal

117 **A.C. Yao, M.H. Kim, A. Gatmaitan, P. Nuchpuckdee and G. Valencia**
Developmental difference in peripheral circulatory response to feeding of newborn and growing preterm infants
Différence de réponse de la circulation périphérique chez le prématuré nouveau-né et en cours d'élevage, selon l'âge conceptionnel

125 **G. Marchini, H. Lagercrant, J. Winberg and K. Uvnäs-Moberg**
Gastrointestinal hormones in newborn infants: release mechanisms and possible circulatory effects
Hormones gastrointestinales chez le nouveau-né humain: mécanismes de libération: effets circulatoires possibles

ONSET OF BREATHING, RESPIRATORY ADAPTATION, SURFACTANT
INSTALLATION DE LA RESPIRATION, ADAPTATION RESPIRATOIRE, SURFACTANT

131 **P. Karlberg and G. Wennergren**
Respiratory control during onset of breathing
Contrôle de la respiration durant son installation néonatale

145 **G. Faxelius, K. Bremme, H. Lagercrantz and J. Milerad**
Respiratory adaptation and hormonal surge at birth: possible sex differences
Adaptation respiratoire et poussée hormonale néonatale: différences peut-être liées au sexe

153 **H. Lagercrantz, B.B. Fredholm, L. Irestedt, M. Runold and A. Sollevi**
Adenosine—a neuromodulator released during asphyxia and a mediator of some hypoxic effects in the newborn?
L'adénosine est-elle un neuromédiateur libéré pendant l'asphyxie, responsable de certains effets liés à l'hypoxie chez le nouveau-né?

161 **J.B. Warshaw, S. Jamieson and J. Sissom**
Factors influencing surfactant synthesis and release
Facteurs jouant un rôle dans la synthèse et la libération du surfactant

173 **L. Marin, F. Dameron, M.E. Dufour and N. Guettari**
Differentiation of type II pneumonocytes in immature rat lung studied by means of intra-embryonic grafting and *in vitro* culture
Différenciation des pneumonocytes de type II dans le poumon de rat immature: étude menée par greffes intra-embryonnaires et cultures in vitro

PERINATAL PHARMACOLOGY
PHARMACOLOGIE PERINATALE

185 **L.O. Boréus**
John Lind and perinatal pharmacology
John Lind et la pharmacologie périnatale

DEDICATION TO JOHN LIND
EN HOMMAGE A JOHN LIND

195 **J. Metcoff**
Space, form and illusion
L'espace, la forme et l'illusion

203 List of participants
Liste des participants

John Lind 1909–1983

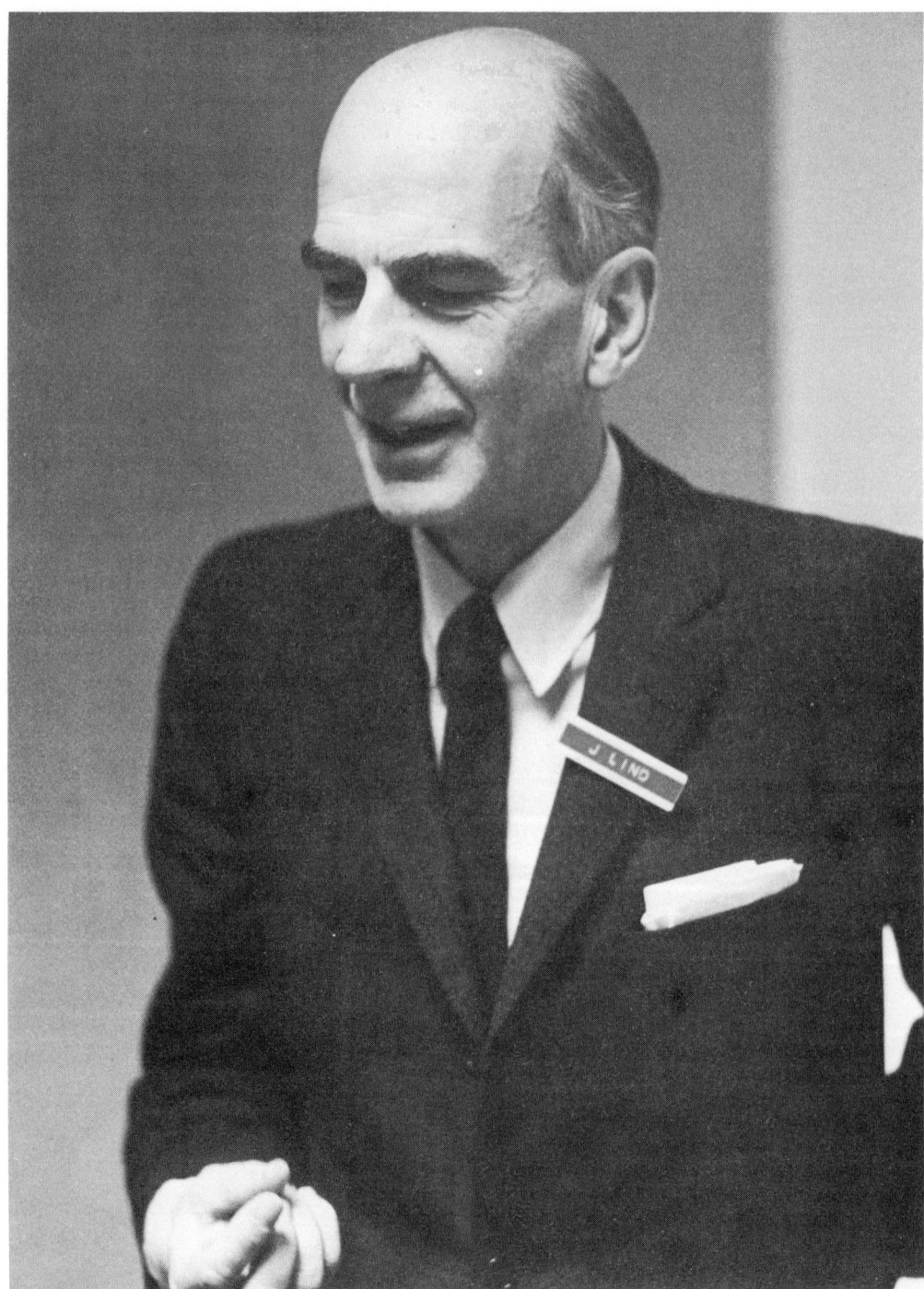

John Lind 1909–1983

John Lind was born in Stockholm in 1909 and received his education and medical school training in that city. In 1950 he was awarded the M.D. Degree from the Karolinska Institute for his thesis on the subject of "Heart Volume in Normal Infants: A Roentgenologic Study", an event which signaled his interest in the then newly developing area of angiocardiography as a tool for the understanding of the normal and abnormal fetal and neonatal circulation and its use as a diagnostic aid in the delineation of various forms of congenital heart disease in children. For the next eight years he was a fulltime Research Investigator at the Wenner-Gren Cardiovascular Research Laboratory whose direction he had assumed in 1955. Coupled with this was a post as Consultant Pediatrician to the Southern Maternity Hospital (Sodra BB) in Stockholm, a position which he had actually held for five years previous to the completion of his M.D. thesis. It was in these two locales that Dr. Lind developed his research activities and in which the many overseas trainees who were subsequently to work with him were nurtured.

Dr. Lind's pioneering studies followed the early animal experiments of Barclay, Franklin, and Pritchard in Great Britain, who had themselves expanded the work of Sir Joseph Barcroft. Recognition of Professor Lind's logical extension of these studies to the area of the human fetus and newborn was evident in his being awarded the Barclay Prize by the British Institute of Radiology in 1959, as well as numerous other international awards which have followed since then, among which are the Ylppo Gold Medal for Pediatric Research in Helsinki in 1967, the Silver Medal for Scientific Merit by the Pediatric Society of Argentina in 1974, and the Gold Medal of the Finnish National Heart Association in 1976

In 1957, he was named Professor of Pediatrics at the Karolinska Institute in Stockholm and Head of the Children's Clinic at the Institute's Hospital. He held this position for more than 20 years, during which time he maintained both the Cardiovascular Research Laboratory at Norrtull's Hospital and the Research Department in the maternity hospital with which he was associated. It is the period of time immediately preceding his acceptance of the Professorship and the years ensuing that proved to be so fertile a period, not only for him, but also for the many international colleagues and trainees who had the privilege of working with him.

It can be said that the impact an individual makes on science and society relates to that which he does and also to that which those who have learned their craft from him subsequently accomplish. In this regard Dr Lind was an individual of outstanding merit, not only in his own right as reflected by his international recognition in the area of neonatal cardiopulmonary physiology, but also in the reputations and achievements of those who were his students His own recognition as Guest Lecturer on both sides of the Atlantic in a number of institutions and medical schools was matched only by his international memberships in pediatric societies which included, in addition to the Scandinavian ones, the Pediatric Societies of France, Switzerland, Portugal, Great Britain, and the United States, as well as those of Austria and Brazil. He was, in addition, an honorary member of the European Club of Pediatrics, the British Neonatal Society and a Board member of the World Federation of Mental Health.

Professor Lind's institute and laboratories were, for a period of over 30 years, filled by fellows and research trainees from many countries and continents. It is a lasting tribute to his impact and influence as a scientist and human being that all of them remember not only the science he taught but also the intense humanism that accompanied these instructions. A research fellow fortunate enough to work in his group would have obtained an excellent introduction to the methodology and thought processes of perinatal physiology and also an appreciation of art, music, literature, and those things that are important to the overall spectrum of human social existence.

The research laboratory at Norrtull's Hospital displayed a large map of the world with many pins and colored indicators of the countries of origin of those who had trained there. At first glance, many of the places seemed exotic and far away. It is a tribute to the quality of the environment that Professor Lind created in bringing together individuals from many different places, that all of the places seemed close, important, and clearly interrelated in the service of humanity and the care of children.

Following his retirement from the Chair of Pediatrics in 1976, Professor Lind pursued studies and research in other directions. His interest in parent-infant interrelations, particularly in the role of the father in the perinatal environment, led him to studies of the responses of the newborn to society, and into such areas as fetal and neonatal perception, studies of the infant cry, and perinatal behaviour. He continued to bring out the best in science and medicine, just as his trainees and colleagues continued to appreciate him as a scientist, a humanist, and most of all as a close and valued friend.

John Lind died in Stockholm, a city he loved so well, on the 8th of January 1983. Tempered with our sadness is our thankfulness both for his life and its contribution to children, as well as for the opportunity of having known him.

Leo Stern, M.D.

John Lind Memorial Lecture
Conférence d'ouverture en hommage à John Lind

Venous return and cardiac output in the perinatal period

A.M. Rudolph

Cardiovascular Research Institute and the Departments of Pediatrics, Physiology, and Obstetrics, Gynecology, and Reproductive Sciences, University of California, San Francisco, and Mount Zion Hospital, San Francisco, California, USA

ABSTRACT

During fetal life, oxygenation occurs in the placenta and oxygenated blood returns to the fetal body in the umbilical veins. Umbilical venous return accounts for about 40% of combined ventricular output. About half the umbilical venous blood passes through the hepatic circulation and the remainder passes through the ductus venosus directly to the inferior vena cava. The left and right lobes of the liver have different blood supplies, resulting in differences in oxygen saturation in hepatic venous blood. Preferential streaming of oxygenated and systemic venous blood in the inferior vena cava is important in providing oxygen and energy substrate supply to the fetal heart and brain. The fetal myocardium is morphologically and functionally immature and the fetal heart appears to be performing near the top of its function curve, so that increasing filling pressure produces limited increase in ventricular output. After birth, left ventricular output increases dramatically, and resting output is high in relation to body weight. With advancing postnatal age, cardiac output falls in relation to body weight, but increases progressively in relation to resting levels, indicating greater reserve. The increase in cardiac output and myocardial performance in the early neonatal period appears to be the result of thyroid hormone activity in late prenatal life.

KEY WORDS

Fetal circulation, hepatic blood flow, ductus venosus, cardiac output regulation, thyroid hormone

INTRODUCTION

John Lind made important contributions to many aspects of perinatology and pediatrics. Early in his career, he examined blood flow patterns in human fetuses, using angiographic techniques. These studies corroborated that the patterns of flow observed in human fetuses were similar to those in fetal lambs, and stimulated my interest in the fetal circulation. I am indeed privileged to pay tribute to John Lind, for whom I have always had admiration and respect. In this presentation I plan to review progress made in the 30-35 years after John Lind's investigations on fetal flow patterns.

In the mammalian fetus, blood is oxygenated in the placenta and the oxygenated blood returns to the fetus through the umbilical veins to the hepatic portal sinus. The portal vein, draining the spleen and gastrointestinal tract, also drains into the portal sinus, so that the venous blood can mix with oxygenated blood at this site. From the portal sinus, blood can either enter the hepatic circulation, or bypass the liver through the ductus venosus to pass directly into the inferior vena cava (Fig. 1). In the inferior vena cava, just below the diaphragm, four streams of blood converge: blood from the distal (abdominal) inferior vena cava, from the left and right hepatic veins, and from the ductus venosus. Inferior vena caval blood can then pass either through the foramen ovale into the left atrium, or through the right atrium and tricuspid valve to the right ventricle. Superior vena caval blood, which constitutes systemic venous blood from the brain and tissues of the head and upper extremities or forelimbs, enters the right atrium and can pass either through the foramen ovale or through the tricuspid valve. Right ventricular blood is ejected into the pulmonary trunk and may enter the pulmonary circulation, or may be diverted away from the lungs through the ductus arteriosus to the descending aorta. In the left atrium, blood coursing through the foramen ovale is joined by pulmonary venous blood and then ejected by the left ventricle into the ascending aorta; the blood is then distributed to the heart through coronary arteries, to the brain, and to the head, neck, and upper extremities. The remainder of the left ventricular blood traverses the aortic isthmus to the descending aorta. Descending aortic blood, derived from aortic isthmus and ductus arteriosus flows, is distributed to lower body and extremity tissues, and also to the placenta.

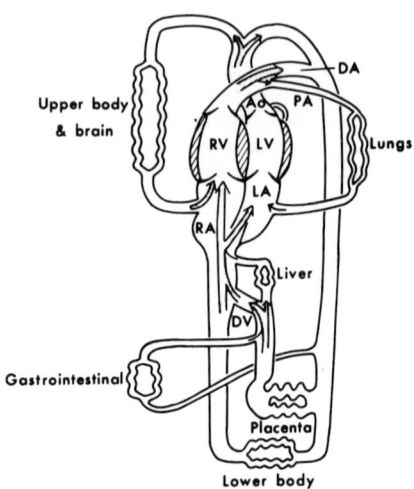

FETAL CIRCULATION

Fig. 1. Diagram of the fetal circulation showing the course of blood flow. DA-ductus arteriosus, Ao-aorta, PA-pulmonary artery, RV-right ventricle, LV-left ventricle, RA-right atrium, LA-left atrium, DV-ductus venosus.

Unlike the adult circulation, in which blood flows sequentially through the systemic and pulmonary circulation, the fetal circulation is designed to permit mixing of oxygenated blood and systemic venous blood. Although the general course of the circulation in the mammalian fetus had been defined by angiographic studies, the actual proportions of venous blood passing through the various shunts have not been delineated. Application of the radionuclide-labeled microsphere method has facilitated studies on the course and distribution of blood derived from different venous channels. In general, studies have been conducted in fetal lambs in utero, to attempt to avoid the effects of acute surgical intervention and of exteriorization of the fetus (Rudolph and Heymann, 1967).

In the adult, with series circulation, cardiac output has been defined as the volume of blood passing through the systemic and pulmonary circulations per unit time. In the fetus, because of the presence of shunts, oxygenated umbilical venous blood and systemic venous blood from the fetal body are distributed to fetal tissues and to the placenta. The definition of cardiac output as defined in the adult cannot be applied, so the term <u>combined ventricular output</u> has been used to describe the output of the two ventricles. It represents all blood distributed to the fetal body and the placenta. By use of the microsphere method, the percentages of combined ventricular output traversing the major fetal vascular channels have been measured in fetal lambs in utero (Heymann et al., 1973). These are shown in Fig. 2. The combined ventricular output in the fetal lamb is about 450-500 ml/min per kg fetal body weight; about 40 percent or 200 ml/min/kg is distributed to the placenta.

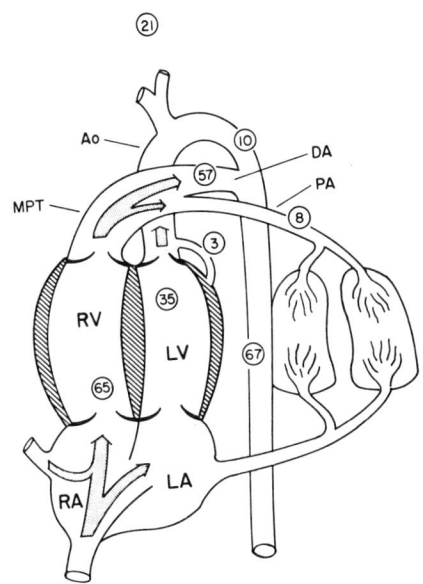

Fig. 2. Diagram of fetal lamb heart showing percentage of combined ventricular output ejected by each ventricle and the proportions passing through main vessels.

Venous Flow Patterns

Superior vena caval blood enters the right atrium and is largely directed across the tricuspid valve into the right ventricle. Only 2-3 percent of superior vena caval blood crosses the foramen ovale; during fetal hypoxemia, this proportion does not change significantly but during umbilical cord compression it increases to about 6 percent (Itskovitz and Rudolph, unpublished observations).

Umbilical venous blood, with an average oxygen saturation of about 85%, enters the portal sinus and is distributed to both lobes of the liver and through the ductus venosus. Under resting conditions in the fetal lamb in utero, about 45 percent passes into the hepatic microcirculation and 55 percent flows through the ductus venosus, but there is considerable variation among fetuses. Portal venous blood, with an O_2 saturation of about 30 percent, is directed almost entirely into the hepatic circulation and only small amounts pass through the ductus venosus (Edelstone and Rudolph, 1979; Bristow et al., 1983). The distribution of blood within the liver is of considerable interest. It had generally been thought that portal and umbilical venous blood mix in the portal sinus and are then distributed to the liver and ductus venosus. Angiographic studies by Lind (1963) in human fetuses demonstrated the morphologic arrangement of the vessels in the porta hepatis, and this has been shown to be similar in fetal lambs (Fig. 3) (Edelstone and Rudolph, 1979; Bristow et al., 1981). The umbilical vein provides branches to the left lobe of the liver, then gives rise to the ductus venosus, after which it arches to the right and joins the portal vein. The left lobe of the liver receives branches from the portal sinus region beyond the junction of the umbilical and portal veins.

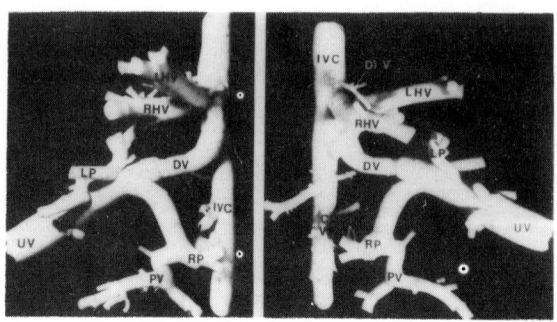

Fig. 3. Silicone rubber cast showing vessels in region of the liver in the fetal lamb, viewed from the left (left) and the right (right) sides. LHV, RHV-left and right hepatic veins, DV-ductus venosus, IVC-inferior vena cava, DiV-diaphragmatic vein, LP, RP-left and right portal venous branches to liver, UV-umbilical vein, PV-portal vein. (From Bristow et al., 1981.)

Blood flow in the porta hepatis is patterned by this morphological arrangement (Fig. 4). The left lobe of the liver receives blood almost exclusively from the umbilical vein, with only a small proportion from the hepatic artery; no portal venous blood passes to the left lobe. The right lobe receives blood from the umbilical vein, and almost all the portal venous blood is directed into the right lobe of the liver. Less than 5 percent of portal venous blood passes through the ductus venosus. The hepatic arterial blood supply to the right lobe is also small. The blood flows per unit of weight of liver tissues do not differ greatly between the left and right lobes, although the flow to the right lobe is somewhat higher.

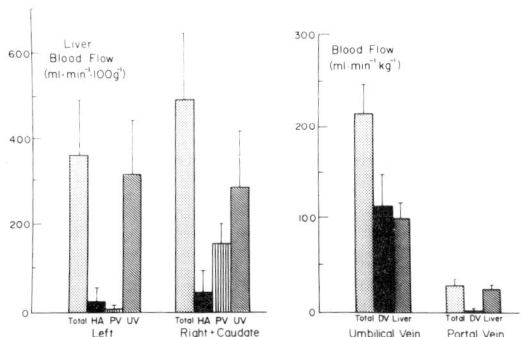

Fig. 4. Left panel - Blood flow in relation to liver tissue weight and the source of blood from the hepatic artery (HA), portal vein (PV), and umbilical vein (UV) is shown to left and right liver lobes. Right panel - Distribution of umbilical venous and portal venous flows to the liver and through the ductus venosus (DV) is shown. (From Rudolph, 1983.)

The blood flow patterns in the liver are of potential importance in regulating venous return to the heart, as well as in distributing oxygen and energy substrates to fetal tissues. Umbilical and portal venous blood represents 45-50 percent of the total venous return to the fetal lamb heart, an amount of 220-250 ml/min/kg fetal body weight. Since about half of this normally passes through the ductus venosus, and the other half through the liver, changes in vascular resistances in the hepatic circulation or in the ductus venosus could influence not only the relative proportions of blood passing through the ductus venosus or liver, but also the actual blood flows and thus venous return to the heart. The factors regulating distribution of blood flow through the ductus venosus and the liver have not been fully defined. A sphincter has been described at the origin of the ductus venosus from the umbilical vein (Chacko and Reynolds, 1953); this is evident in Fig. 3.

Edelstone (1980) has suggested that, during fetal life, the ductus venosus responds passively to the pressure within the lumen, and that it does not actively regulate flow. During fetal hypoxemia induced by administering a low oxygen gas mixture to the maternal ewe, umbilical blood flow is maintained, but the proportion passing through the ductus venosus is increased from the control of about 55 percent, to about 65 percent, whilst the porportion entering the liver is reduced to 35 percent. This redistribution could result from relaxation of the ductus venosus sphincter, or from an increase in vascular resistance in the liver; the mechanism has not been fully defined. Vagal stimulation may cause hepatic vasoconstriction during hypoxemia as suggested by studies with acetylcholine, which, when infused into the portal vein, is distributed to the right liver lobe. This markedly reduces blood flow to the right liver lobe, indicating selective vasoconstriction in the hepatic microcirculation (Edelstone et al., 1980).

The distribution of umbilical venous blood between the liver and ductus venosus is also altered by changes in total umbilical blood flow. Reducing umbilical blood flow by inflating a balloon in the descending aorta markedly increases the proportion of umbilical venous blood passing through the ductus venosus and decreases liver blood flow (Edelstone et al., 1980). The total blood flows to the left and right lobes are reduced by similar amounts in relation to tissue weight, but the right lobe receives very little umbilical venous blood, and derives most of its blood supply from the portal vein. Oxygen delivery to the right lobe is therefore drastically reduced (unpublished observations). When umbilical blood flow falls as a result of reduction of blood volume by hemorrhage, hepatic blood flow is reduced, and umbilical venous blood is preferentially distributed through the ductus venosus (Itskovitz et al., 1982).

Ductus venosus blood has an oxygen saturation almost identical with that of umbilical venous blood, because only a small amount of portal venous blood enters the ductus venosus. The ductus venosus enters the inferior vena cava just distal to the diaphragm; the hepatic veins also drain into the inferior vena cava at this site. We felt it was important to determine the oxygen uptake by the liver, and the distribution of oxygenated umbilical venous blood and of systemic venous blood. We developed techniques to catheterize fetal hepatic veins and to monitor catheters in the umbilical, portal, and hepatic veins chronically in utero (Bristow et al., 1981). Because the blood supplies of the left and right lobes of the liver are different, whereas oxygen consumption of each lobe in relation to tissue weight is similar, the oxygen saturation of the left hepatic vein is higher than that of the right. Left hepatic venous O_2 saturation is about 8-10 percent lower than that in the umbilical vein, whereas right hepatic venous saturation is similar to that in the descending aorta (about 55 percent). To assess the distribution of the four blood streams with different oxygen saturations, which join in the inferior vena cava just distal to the diaphragm, we used the radionuclide-labeled microsphere technique.

When microspheres with different labels were injected simultaneously into the umbilical venous and distal (abdominal) inferior vena caval streams, it was evident that umbilical venous blood was preferentially directed across the foramen ovale to be distributed to the upper body organs, including the myocardium and brain; distal inferior vena caval blood passed preferentially across the tricuspid valve to the right ventricle and then through the pulmonary trunk and ductus arteriosus to the descending aorta and lower body organs. When microspheres are injected into the umbilical vein, those that reach the hepatic circulation are trapped in the liver; thus the preferential streaming across the foramen ovale represents the distribution of spheres that passed through the ductus venosus. From studies in which microspheres were injected into the left or right hepatic veins it was demonstrated that blood from these veins also shows streaming patterns in the thoracic inferior vena cava. Right hepatic venous blood, with an oxygen saturation lower than that in the left hepatic vein, is preferentially directed in a similar manner to distal inferior vena caval blood through the tricuspid valve, whereas left hepatic venous blood follows the distribution of ductus venosus blood. The patterns of venous blood flow in the liver and heart are summarized in Fig. 5.

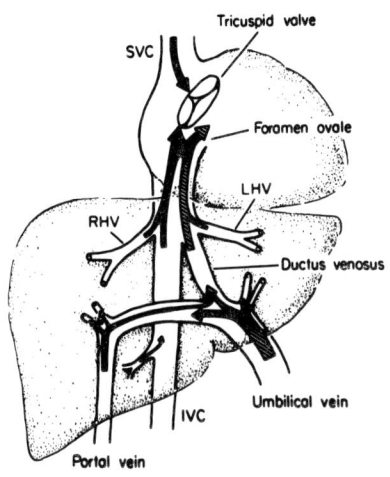

Fig. 5. Patterns of blood flow in the fetal liver and in the thoracic inferior vena cava, as described in text. (From Rudolph, 1983.)

The mechanisms responsible for the preferential streaming of blood entering the inferior vena cava have not been fully elucidated. Inspection of the thoracic portion of the inferior vena cava in the fetal lamb reveals the presence of a stream of well-oxygenated blood in the dorsal and leftward position of the vessel, and a stream of poorly-oxygenated blood in the ventral and rightward region. The morphology of this region could contribute to the flow patterns. In the fetal lamb, the left hepatic vein and ductus venosus join immediately before connecting with the inferior vena cava (Fig. 3). A thin translucent valve-like structure covers the joint orifice of the left hepatic vein and ductus venosus, attached along the distal margin. A similar membrane covers the distal portion of the orifice of the right hepatic vein. We have suggested that these membranes direct the blood streams, as they enter the inferior vena cava, to produce the preferential distribution patterns (Bristow et al., 1981). The streaming patterns of blood could also be influenced by hemodynamic changes, such as alterations in velocity of flow in either the ductus venosus or inferior vena cava, or changes in hepatic and ductus venosus flow relationships, but this has not as yet been examined.

The streamlining of blood in the fetal circulation has important effects on the distribution of oxygen and energy substrates to fetal tissues (Edelstone and Rudolph, 1979; Reuss et al., 1981). The higher oxygen saturation of ascending aortic blood (about 65 percent) as compared with descending aortic blood (about 55 percent) results from the passage of almost all superior vena caval blood through the tricuspid valve into the right ventricle, as well as from the preferential distribution of the various blood streams entering the vena cava. Furthermore, energy substrates delivered to the fetus from placental passage from the maternal circulation into the umbilical vein, would also be present in higher concentrations in the ascending aorta. This has been shown for glucose (Charlton and Johengen, 1984). The effect of these flow patterns is to deliver blood with higher oxygen content and substrate concentrations to the brain and heart, which have high metabolic activity in the fetus, and blood with lower oxygen content to the descending aorta, from which most of the blood passes to the placenta, where oxygenation occurs.

Fetal Cardiac Output
As has been mentioned above, because of mixing of oxygenated and systemic venous blood entering the heart, and the apparently parallel rather than series nature of the ventricles, it has become customary to consider the cardiac output in the fetus as combined ventricular output of both ventricles. In the adult mammal, the stroke volumes of the two ventricles are almost identical. In the fetal lamb, the right ventricle is dominant and ejects about 66 percent of combined ventricular output, whereas the right ventricle ejects 34 percent.

Ventricular output is the product of heart rate and stroke volume. We examined the effects of heart rate changes in chronically-instrumented fetal lambs, in which an electromagnetic flow transducer was applied around the aorta or pulmonary trunk to measure left and right ventricular volumes. Spontaneous changes in heart rate were noted to produce consistent alterations in left and right ventricular output. Increases in heart rate above the resting levels were associated with small increases in both left and right ventricular output. The stroke volume of each ventricle fell with increasing heart rates, but the output of each ventricle increased by about 10-15 percent above baseline levels, as heart rates increased to 240-270 beats per minute. Spontaneous decreases in heart rate were associated with only small increases in stroke volume, so that when the rate fell spontaneously below about 150 beats per minute, ventricular output fell progressively with the decline in heart rate (Rudolph and Heymann, 1976). When heart rate was increased above resting levels by pacing the left atrium, right ventricular output increased by a maximum of about 10-15 percent, but left ventricular output fell markedly. The fall in left ventricular output with left atrial pacing could be related to abnormal atrial pressure contours, so that, with the abnormal origin of the atrial impulse, the pressure relationships between the inferior vena cava and right and left atrium were altered, thus interfering with flow across the foramen ovale, and filling of the left ventricle. Reducing heart rate by stimulating the cervical portion of the vagus nerve resulted in a dramatic fall in both right and left ventricular outputs.

From these studies, it is evident that although the fetal ventricles can increase stroke volume, their ability to do so is limited, so that cardiac output cannot be maintained when heart rate falls significantly below resting levels. The reason for this restriction in ability to increase stroke volume could be related to several factors, including an inability to maintain output with increased afterload or outflow resistance, inadequate preload or filling pressure, poor compliance of the ventricular muscle, and poor intrinsic myocardial contractility.

Studies on the output of the left and right ventricles and their responses to alterations in afterload suggest that differences in afterload are largely responsible for the markedly higher right than left ventricular output in the fetal lamb. The velocity patterns recorded simultaneously by electromagnetic flow transducers around the ascending aorta and pulmonary trunk show several differences in the two vessels. The larger area under the velocity tracing from the pulmonary trunk confirms the greater right ventricular stroke volume. There is a more rapid acceleration in the pulmonary trunk, and greater backflow just prior to semilunar valve closure in the ascending aorta. These differences suggest that, since the two ventricles have similar filling pressures and are ejecting at essentially the same pressures, the left ventricle is presented with a larger outflow resistance than the right ventricle, and that the aortic isthmus is the site of functional separation of the circulation (Fig. 2). The left ventricle can be considered to be ejecting into the ascending aorta and the circulations of the head and forelimbs, whereas the right ventricle ejects largely through the ductus arteriosus into the descending aorta to the lower body and umbilical-placental circulations. To demonstrate that there is functional separation at the aortic isthmus, we injected small bolus amounts of norepinephrine to produce vasoconstriction, or acetylcholine to cause vasodilatation, into the ascending or descending aorta. When injected into the descending aorta, acetylcholine resulted in a greater fall in descending than ascending aortic pressure for several beats; when acetylcholine was injected into the ascending aorta, ascending aortic pressure fell more than descending aortic pressure. Furthermore, when acetylcholine was injected into the descending aorta, right ventricular stroke volume increased for several beats, but left ventricular stroke volume did not change. When norepinephrine was injected into the ascending or descending aorta, greater increases in pressure were observed for several beats in the circulation into which it was injected (unpublished observations). To summarize these observations, it is suggested that the fetal circulation is functionally separated by the aortic isthmus, the portion of the aorta just above the ductus arteriosus; the left ventricle has a relatively high afterload of the upper body circulation and the aortic isthmus, and therefore a lower stroke volume, whereas the right ventricle has a lower afterload of the lower body and umbilical-placental circulation, and a higher stroke volume.

The role of preload, or filling pressure, of the ventricles in determining ventricular stroke volume has been studied by several investigators. We found that rapid infusions of saline into fetal lambs increased right ventricular output only slightly, even though ventricular end-diastolic pressure increased markedly (Heymann and Rudolph, 1973). Similar observations were reported by Gilbert (1982) who showed that reducing right atrial pressure by hemorrhage caused a marked fall in combined ventricular output, but volume infusions, which markedly increased right atrial pressure, resulted in only small increases in output when raised above the resting levels of 3-5 mmHg. Using electromagnetic flow transducers for measuring cardiac output, Thornburg and Morton (1983) have reported similar results. In all these studies the ventricular function curves were obtained by relating cardiac output or stroke volume to atrial or ventricular end-diastolic pressure. However, the Frank-Starling relationship is based on the resting or diastolic length of the muscle fiber and therefore depends on end-diastolic volume rather than end-diastolic pressure.

The compliance of the ventricles is important in determining the volume at any filling pressure. Thus if the ventricle is relatively stiff, it would not be easily distended, even if filling pressure is relatively high. The fetal lamb ventricle has been shown to be much less compliant than that of the newborn lamb, which in turn is less compliant than the adult heart (Romero et al., 1972). Thus the relatively flat ventricular function curve above end-diastolic pressures of 4-5 mmHg could be related to the poor compliance of the fetal ventricle, rather than limited myocardial function.

Cardiac Output after Birth
Measurements in lambs after birth have shown that cardiac output increases (Lister et al., 1979; Edelstone et al., 1980). Although right ventricular output increases only modestly from the fetal level of 300 ml/kg/min to 350-400 ml/kg/min, left ventricular output increases dramatically from the fetal level of 150 ml/kg/min to 350-400 ml/kg/min, a 2 to 2-1/2 fold rise. Following this early increase, the cardiac output falls progressively in relation to body weight, so that by 6 weeks after birth, the output has fallen to about 160 ml/kg/min. The high output during the first weeks of life is partly related to the marked increase in oxygen consumption after birth, associated with increased metabolic

activity necessary for maintenance of body temperature. In the lamb, oxygen
consumption during fetal life is about 7-8 ml/kg body weight/min and this
increases to about 14-18 ml/kg/min after birth. During the next 6 weeks it falls
to about 10 ml/kg/min. The changes in oxygen consumption alone cannot account
for the alterations of cardiac output. During fetal life, about 38 ml blood is
required to provide 1 ml oxygen consumption. This falls to about 28 ml/ml VO_2
after birth. This initial change is related to the increase in oxygen saturation
and oxygen content of arterial blood after birth, so that less blood flow is
necessary to provide the same oxygen delivery. Subsequently, there is a further
fall in the cardiac output required to provide oxygen, and the blood flow/VO_2
ratio falls to about 15 ml/ml VO_2. This later change can be related to the
change in hemoglobin from the fetal to adult type over the 6-8 weeks after
birth. Fetal blood has a P50 of 38 torr. Postnatally, arterial blood has a
PO_2 of 95-100 torr, and venous blood a PO_2 of 35-40 torr. The slope of the
oxygen equilibration curves would therefore permit larger quantities of oxygen to
be extracted per unit volume of blood in the presence of adult as compared with
fetal hemoglobin (Fig. 6).

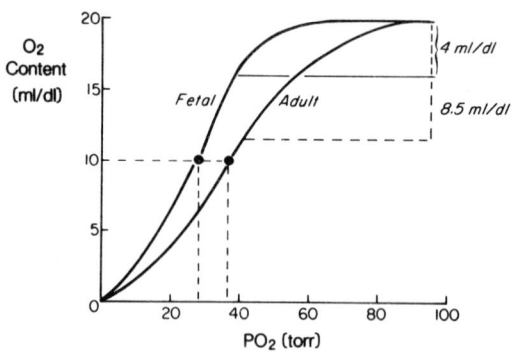

Fig. 6. Diagram showing effect of change of hemoglobin
from fetal to adult type on oxygen availability
postnatally. With arterial PO_2 of 95 and venous PO_2
of 40 torr, 4 ml/dl of blood would be extracted from
fetal hemoglobin, but 8.5 ml/dl from adult hemoglobin.

Because cardiac output is very high in relation to body weight in the early
neonatal period, we wished to assess whether it could be increased further and
studied the effects of rapid infusions of saline to increase preload in
chronically-instrumented lambs (Klopfenstein and Rudolph, 1978). In the first
week after birth, cardiac output could be raised by about 35 percent above
resting levels; by 6-8 weeks after birth, it could be increased by 65 percent
above control values. This indicated that there was a high resting level of
cardiac output in the early neonatal period, but a limited reserve to further
increase output, whereas later, resting output requirements in relation to body
weight fell, but circulatory reserve was greater. Recent studies in our
laboratory have shown that intrinsic myocardial contractility is very high in the
neonatal lamb, and progressively falls during the first 6 weeks. However, there
is minimal response of contractility to isoproterenol during the first postnatal
week; the response increases over the next 4-6 weeks (Teitel et al., 1985).
Those studies tended to corroborate the previous observations that circulatory
performance is excellent but reserve is limited.

It is of interest that in the fetal lamb, ventricular output cannot be increased by more than 20-25 percent with maximal volume loading, yet after birth, left ventricular output increases spontaneously by 100 percent or more and further increases can develop with volume loading. This change could be related to increased sympathetico-adrenal activity after birth, because plasma catecholamine concentrations have been shown to increase (Padbury et al., 1981). However, administration of beta-adrenergic blockers to newborn lambs produced a small decrease in cardiac output, but did not lower cardiac output to fetal levels. We considered the possibility that the rise in plasma thyroid hormone concentrations after birth could influence myocardial performance and thereby account for the increased cardiac output after birth.

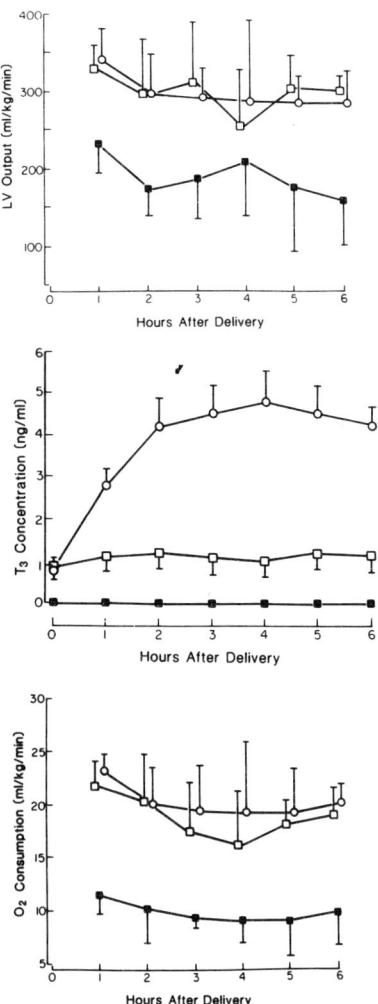

Fig. 7. Changes in left ventricular output, plasma triiodothyronine (T_3) concentrations, and oxygen consumption after birth in normal lambs ○ , lambs subjected to thyroidectomy about 2 weeks prior to delivery ■ , and lambs subjected to thyroidectomy immediately before delivery □ .

We prepared three groups of fetal lambs at about 130 days gestation and measured left ventricular outputs and oxygen consumptions after delivery by cesarean section almost 2 weeks later. The first group served as control; the second group had thyroidectomy performed at the time of the original surgery; the third group had thyroidectomy performed just prior ro cesarean section (Breall et al., 1984). In the control group, plasma triiodothyronine (T_3) concentrations increased rapidly after delivery, and oxygen consumption and left ventricular output were high (Fig. 7). The lambs that had thyroidectomy performed at delivery showed no rise in plasma T_3 concentrations, but oxygen consumption and left ventricular output values were similar to those observed in the normal lambs. Lambs that had thyroidectomy 2 weeks before delivery had low plasma T_3 concentrations that did not increase after delivery. These lambs also showed low oxygen consumption and left ventricular output values that were not much higher than those we have measured during fetal life; furthermore, they had low heart rates as compared with the other two groups. These studies indicate that thyroid hormone is important in maturation of the heart and in the postnatal increase in cardiac output as well as oxygen consumption. However, it is not the postnatal rise in plasma T_3 concentrations, but rather the influence of thyroid in the latter days of gestation, that results in myocardial maturational changes. The exact mechanisms by which this change is accomplished have not been defined. Thyroid hormones are known to have many effects on heart muscle including Na^+K^+ATPase activity (Philipson and Edelman, 1977), cardiac myosin ATPase activity (Morkin, 1979), and beta-adrenergic receptor activity (Whitsett et al., 1982). We are currently investigating the possibility that thyroid hormone increases beta-adrenergic receptor numbers or function in the fetal myocardium.

Our current concept concerning the perinatal changes in cardiac performance is shown in Fig. 8. During fetal life the myocardium has a relatively poor contractility and is performing near the top of its function curve, so that, although ventricular output falls when filling pressure is reduced below its resting level of 3-5 mmHg, increasing filling pressure above this level produces only a modest increase in output. After birth, myocardial contractility increases markedly, possibly as a result of sympathetico-adrenal stimulation. The increase in myocardial contractility is, however, dependent on prenatal thyroid effect. However, because the resting cardiac output requirements are so high, reserve is limited, as is the ability to increase output further. With postnatal development, the resting output requirements fall in relation to body weight, but myocardial reserve progressively increases.

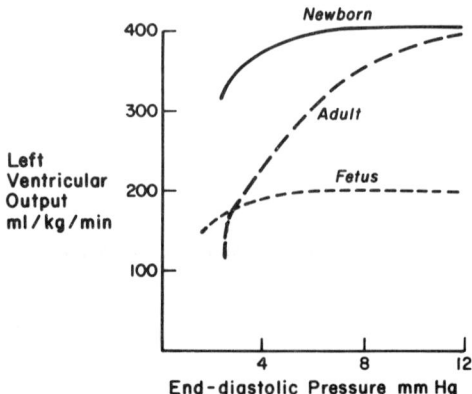

Fig. 8. Diagram showing concept of changes in left ventricular output at different filling pressures, at different periods of development, as described in text.

REFERENCES

Breall, J.A., Rudolph, A.M., Heymann M.A. (1984): Role of thyroid hormone in postnatal circulatory and metabolic adjustments. J. Clin. Invest. 73, 1418-1424.

Bristow, J., Rudolph, A.M., Itskovitz, J. (1981): A preparation for studying liver blood flow, oxygen consumption, and metabolism in the fetal lamb in utero. J. Dev. Physiol. 3, 255-266.

Bristow, J., Rudolph, A.M, Itskovitz, J., Barnes, R.J. (1983): Hepatic oxygen and glucose metabolism in the fetal lamb: Response to hypoxia. J. Clin. Invest. 71, 1047-1061.

Chacko, G.F. Jr., Reynolds, S.R.M. (1953): Embryonic development in the human of the sphincter of the ductus venosus. Anat. Record. 115, 151-173.

Charlton, V., Johengen, M. (1984): Nutrient and waste product concentration differencs in fetal upper and lower body arteries. J. Dev. Physiol. 6, 431-437.

Edelstone, D.I. (1980): Regulation of blood flow through the ductus venosus. J. Dev. Physiol. 2, 219-238.

Edelstone, D.I., Rudolph, A.M. (1979): Preferential streaming of ductus venosus blood to the brain and heart in fetal lambs. Am. J. Physiol. 237, H724-H729.

Edelstone, D.I., Rudolph, A.M., Heymann, M.A. (1978): Liver and ductus venosus blood flows in fetal lambs in utero. Circ. Res. 42, 426-433.

Edelstone, D.I., Rudolph, A.M., Heymann, M.A. (1980): Effects of hypoxemia and decreasing umbilical flow on liver and ductus venosus blood flows in fetal lambs. Am. J. Physiol 238, H656-H663.

Gilbert, R.D. (1982): Effects of afterload and baroreceptors on cardiac function in fetal sheep. J. Dev. Physiol. 4, 299-309.

Heymann, M.A., Creasy, R.K., Rudolph, A.M. (1973): Quantitation of blood flow pattern in foetal lamb in utero. In Proceedings of the Sir Joseph Barcroft Centenary Symposium: Foetal and Neonatal Physiology, pp 89-111. Cambridge: Cambridge University Press.

Heymann, M.A., Rudolph, A.M. (1973): Effects of increasing preload on right ventricular output in fetal lambs in utero (abstr). Circulation 48, (Suppl IV):37.

Itskovitz, J., Goetzman, B., Rudolph, A.M. (1982): Effects of hemorrhage on umbilical venous return and oxygen delivery in fetal lambs. Am. J. Physiol. 242, H543-H548.

Klopfenstein, H.S., Rudolph, A.M. (1978): Postnatal changes in the circulation, and responses to volume loading in sheep. Circ. Res. 42, 839-845.

Lind, J. (1963): Changes in the liver circulation at birth. Ann. N.Y. Acad. Sci. 111, 110-120.

Lister, G., Walter, T.K., Versmold, H.T., Dallman, P.R., Rudolph, A.M. (1979): Oxygen delivery in lambs: Cardiovascular and hematologic development. Am. J. Physiol. 237, H668-H675.

Morkin, E. (1979): Stimulation of cardiac myosin adenosine triphosphatase in thyrotoxicosis. Circ. Res. 44, 1-7.

Padbury, J.F., Diakomanolis, E.S., Hobel, C.J., Perelman, A., Fisher, D.A. (1981): Neonatal adaptation: Sympatho-adrenal response to cord cutting. Pediatr. Res. 15, 1483-1487.

Philipson, K.D., Edelman, I.S. (1977): Thyroid hormone control of Na^+, K^+-ATPase and K^+-dependent phosphatase in rat heart. Am. J. Physiol. 232, C196-C206.

Reuss, M.L., Rudolph, A.M., Heymann, M.A. (1981): Selective distribution of microspheres injected into the umbilical veins and inferior venae cavae of fetal sheep. Am. J. Obstet. Gynecol. 141, 427-432.

Romero, T.E., Covell, J., Friedman, W.F. (1972): A comparison of pressure-volume relations of the fetal, newborn, and adult heart. Am. J. Physiol. 222, 1285-1290.

Rudolph, A.M. (1983): Hepatic and ductus venosus blood flows during fetal life. Hepatology 3, 254-258.

Rudolph, A.M., Heymann, M.A. (1967): The circulation of the fetus in utero. Circ. Res. 21, 163-184.

Rudolph, A.M., Heymann, M.A. (1976): Cardiac output in the fetal lamb: The effects of spontaneous and induced changes of heart rate on right and left ventricular output. Am. J. Obstet. Gynecol. 124, 183-192.

Teitel, D., Sidi, D., Chin, T., Brett, C., Heymann, M.A., Rudolph, A.M., Padbury, J.F., Diakomanolis, E.S. (1985): Developmental changes in myocardial contractile reserve in the lamb. Pediatr. Res. (In Press).

Thornburg, K.L., Morton, M.J. (1983): Filling and arterial pressures as determinants of RV stroke volume in the sheep fetus. Am. J. Physiol. 244, H656-H663.

Whitsett, J.A., Noguchi, A., Moore, J.J. (1982): Developmental aspects of alpha- and ß-adrenergic receptors. Semin. Perinatol. 6, 125-141.

This work was supported by grants from the United States Public Health Service, Program Project Grant HL24056 and HL23681.

RESUME.

Il y a 30-35 ans, en utilisant des techniques angiographiques, John Lind a montré que les circuits vasculaires du foetus humain étaient semblables à ceux observés chez le foetus d'agneau. Depuis lors, de nombreuses investigations ont été conduites sur la circulation foetale.

Pendant la vie foetale, l'oxygénation sanguine est réalisée au niveau du placenta et le sang oxygéné retourne au foetus par la veine ombilicale. Le retour veineux ombilical représente environ 40 pour cent du débit ventriculaire total (débit "combiné" des deux ventricules). Environ la moitié du débit veineux ombilical (saturé à 85%) emprunte le canal veineux d'Arantius et se déverse directement dans la veine cave inférieure. Le lobe gauche du foie reçoit presque exclusivement du sang veineux ombilical, tandis que le lobe droit reçoit du sang veineux ombilical mélangé à la quasi-totalité du sang veineux porte (à faible saturation). Moins de 5 pour cent du débit de la veine porte atteint le canal veineux d'Arantius. La consommation en oxygène par unité de tissu hépatique étant similaire dans les deux lobes, la saturation en oxygène de la veine sus-hépatique gauche (environ 75%) est supérieure à celle de la veine sus-hépatique droite (environ 55%). Les courants préférentiels suivis ensuite par le sang oxygéné et le sang veineux systémique jouent un rôle important dans l'apport d'oxygène et de substrats énergétiques au coeur et au cerveau du foetus: le sang veineux ombilical et le sang veineux hépatique gauche passent à travers le foramen ovale et suivent la voie gauche; le sang veineux cave distal et le sang veineux hépatique droit passent en majeure partie à travers la valve tricuspide et suivent la voie droite.

Le myocarde foetal est immature sur le plan fonctionnel aussi bien que morphologique. Le coeur foetal travaille dans un zone proche du sommet de sa courbe fonctionnelle, de telle sorte qu'une augmentation de la pression de remplissage n'entraîne qu'un accroissement limité du débit cardiaque. Après la naissance, le débit ventriculaire gauche s'accroit de façon spectaculaire, et le débit de repos par unité de poids corporel est élevé. Au fur et à mesure que l'âge post-natal augmente, le débit cardiaque rapporté au poids corporel décroit, tout en augmentant progressivement par rapport au débit de repos, ce qui indique l'acquisition d'une plus grande réserve cardiaque.

L'augmentation du débit cardiaque et des performances myocardiques au début de la période néonatale apparait due à l'activité de l'hormone thyroidienne en fin de période prénatale.

****

DISCUSSION. Dr.L.Stern, moderator.

Dr.L.Stern: How do you get from the thyroid to brown fat?

Dr.Ab.Rudolph: Unfortunately, I did not have time to adress this in my presentation. The interest in this relates to studies in which we have found a close relationship between oxygen consumption and cardiac output in newborn lambs (Lister G et al., Amer J Physiol 1979 6:H668). The concept was developed that cardiac output is determined by oxygen consumption. However, many of the events that occur after birth are linked. For example, we know that, in addition to the increase in cardiac output and oxygen consumption, plasma free fatty acid concentrations rise (Van Duyne CM et al., Amer J Physiol 1960; 199:987) and plasma catecholamine concentrations rise. The hypothesis I have been considering is that thyroid hormone, acting prenatally, increases the number or rate of maturation of beta-adrenergic receptors both in the myocardium and in brown fat. It has been shown that thyroid hormone influences myocardial beta-adrenergic receptors (Whitsett JA et al., Pediatr Res 1982; 16:463). Thus, if thyroid hormone increased beta-adrenergic receptor activity in both brown fat and the myocardium, the rise in plasma catecholamines after birth would increase brown fat metabolism (as a result of beta-adrenergic stimulation), increase oxygen consumption, cause a rise in plasma fatty acid concentrations, and increase myocardial performance and heart rate. I hope that answers the question about the relationship between thyroid and brown fat.

Dr.J.Warshaw: Have you looked at T_3 versus T_4 as well as changes in myocardial ultrastructure? Have you examined T_3 binding in reference to other receptors, the beta-receptor for example?

Dr.Ab.Rudolph: We have only recently done the thyroid studies. We have not yet examined whether morphological changes in the myocardium occur in the period immediately prior to birth. Most previous observations on myocardial morphology have been made during an earlier period of fetal life, and these have been compared with morphology in the neonatal and adult periods. We know that plasma concentrations of cortisol in fetal lambs begin to increase from about 125 days gestation and there is a sharp further rise 2-3 days prior to delivery (Rose JC et al., J Clin Invest 1978; 61:424; Nathanielsz P., in Fetal Endocrinology, An Experimental Approach, 1976, Amsterdam, Elsevier). There may be an interrelationship between the rise in cortisol levels and T_3 activity.

Dr.J.Warshaw: Have you looked into arginine vasopressin (AVP) or other strategies that the fetus might employ to get more blood flow to support growth?

Dr.Ab.Rudolph: We are currently examining the effects of vasopressin, angiotensin, catecholamines, and alpha- and beta-adrenergic receptor blockade on the hepatic circulation and distributional changes in flow, but we do not have any definite results as yet. It is important to recognize that the preferential flow patterns may influence concentrations of various substances reaching different parts of the fetal body. Thus drugs entering the fetus through the umbilical circulation will tend to reach the brain and heart in higher concentrations than the fetal lower body organs. Also, gastrointestinal hormones, including insulin, which enter the portal vein will reach the right lobe of the liver in higher concentrations than the left lobe. The possible effects of these factors need to be assessed.

Dr.W.Oh: When did you do the thyroidectomy?

Dr.Ab.Rudolph: At about 128-130 days gestation, well before there would normally be a dramatic rise in T_3 concentrations.

Dr.W.Oh: When people did thyroidectomies in the late sixties, they would get intrauterine growth retarded fetuses.

Dr.Ab.Rudolph: They did the thyroidectomy at a much earlier period of gestation. When we did it at about 130 days gestation, we found no significant difference in fetal weight at delivery, and wool development and other external appearances were normal.

Dr.L.Stern: Would you suggest, from what you have been saying, that the limiting feature in cardiac output is essentially an inability to increase substrate?

Dr.Ab.Rudolph: I feel the two are interrelated. They both are, I think, the result of the same stimulus.

Dr.J.Metcoff: What is the pathway for fetal hepatic glucose production?

Dr.Ab.Rudolph: I think that fetal hepatic glucose production results from glycogenolysis. Glycogen in the fetal liver is probably produced from lactate; we have shown that there is net lactate uptake by the liver in the fetal lamb (Gleason CA et al., J Develop Physiol 1985; 8: in press). Recently, it has been shown in the adult liver that glycogen can be produced from lactate (Newgard CG et al., J Biol Chem 1983; 258:8046).

Fetal and neonatal circulation
Circulation foetale et néonatale

Role of intracardiac streaming upon early cardiac development

Rene A. Arcilla

The University of Chicago, 5825 S. Maryland Avenue, Chicago, Illinois 60637, USA

ABSTRACT

The role of intracardiac streaming upon cardiac morphogenesis and bulbo-ventricular septation was examined in chick embryos. Two experiments were performed: scanning electronmicroscopy (SEM) at H-H stages 16-39 (study I), and methylene blue microangiography (MBM) at H-H stages 14-22 (study II). Injection sites for MBM were 9 peripheral vitelline veins. Two cardiac stream patterns were observed. Type A coursed along cranial segments of primitive atrium and AV canal, and ventrally along primitive ventricle (PV) and bulbus. Type B coursed along caudal segments of primitive atrium and AV canal, and dorsally along PV and bulbus. Both flowed in parallel, i.e., did not spiral, along the PV. The SEM study showed untrabeculated PV at stage 16, beginning trabeculation at distal PV and bulbar region by stage 18-19. Trabeculae became organized into sheets in dorsoventral direction. By stages 26-30, the sheets gradually coalesced, initially at bulbo-ventricular area and later extending to floor of PV, to become muscular interventricular septum (MIVS). Our findings do not support the flow-molding concept of cardiac morphogenesis but instead suggest that early development is intrinsic or programmed.

KEY WORDS

chick embryo, cardiac development, ventricular septal formation, intracardiac streaming, microangiography, scanning electronmicroscopy

INTRODUCTION

Most investigations dealing with cardiac morphogenesis have been conducted on chick embryos. The heart is readily accessible, its stage of development can be accurately identified (Hamburger, Hamilton 1951), and the entire spectrum can be analyzed without the frustrating problems caused by gaps in developmental stages which characterize human embryo collections. Although the stages of cardiogenesis in this model are not necessarily identical to those of man, the developmental mechanisms are probably similar if not identical.

The chick myocardium is initially a network of loosely arranged, functionally autonomous myocytes which become more compact at age 24 to 30 hours (H-H stages

7 to 9) (Hibbs, 1956; Manasek, 1968). Initial contractions of the tubular heart are observed by stage 10, at about the time when cardiac looping is also occurring (Patten, Kramer, 1933). Bloodflow is identified several hours later at stage 12. Cardiac septation occurs much later, with atrial septal formation starting by around stage 16-17 and ventricular septal development by stage 26. There is then a definitive period in early embryonic life when the circulation is maintained by a two-chambered tubular heart devoid of valve structures, with a single venous trunk (common omphalomesenteric trunk) opening into a primitive atrium and a single arterial trunk (truncus arteriosus) arising from a primitive ventricle.

Previous investigators have described two intracardiac streams within the developing heart, based on visual observations of the forward movements of the blood cells (Bremer, 1932; Jafee, 1962; Jafee, 1965). A right-heart stream and a left-heart stream were identified which selectively flowed through the right and left sides of the primitive heart, respectively. Both assumed a spiral course at the conotruncus region, with the right-heart stream proceeding ventrally and leftward to reach the more caudal branchial arches, and the left-heart stream proceeding dorsally and rightward to reach the more cranial arches. Based on these observations, the flow-molding theory was conceived which proposed that the intracardiac streams not only mold the developing heart but also play an important role in promoting septation at the ventricular, bulbar and truncal levels (Bremer, 1932).

The morphogenesis of the interventricular septum is still unsettled. Some investigators have suggested that this structure is originally that portion of the ventricular wall, and adjoining trabeculae, that is interposed between the outpocketing free walls of the primitive ventricle as they expand in response to the molding forces of the intracardiac streams (Streeter, 1948; Chang, 1932). Others have proposed that coalescence of the sponge-like trabeculations within the developing ventricle results in formation of the muscular interventricular septum (Patten, 1951; Morse, 1978). It is a traditional view that septal formation starts at the floor of the primitive ventricle and proceeds cranially during its development. By and large, these studies have consisted of reconstructions of histologic sections which, presumably because of the technics used, may have failed to adequately reproduce the delicate architecture of the early developing heart.

The relationship between circulation, cardiac function and cardiac development during embryonic life remains an attractive subject for research on mechanisms and pathogenesis of cardiac malformations. Our studies along this line have focused on the very early stages of cardiogenesis. In this report, I wish to summarize the results of two related investigations on the chick embryonic heart dealing with: (1) the development of the muscular interventricular septum as analyzed by scanning electronmicroscopy, and (2) microangiographic demonstration of intracardiac flow streaming prior to septal development.

I. Morphogenesis of the interventricular septum

Sixty-two chick embryo hearts were studied over a wide spectrum of cardiac development ranging from H-H stage 16 to stage 39. These included stages 12-13 (n=3), stages 17-19 (n=14), stages 20-26 (n=21), stages 27-29 (n=13), stages 30-39 (n=11). Fertilized White Leghorn eggs were incubated at $38°C$ to $39°C$ at constant humidity. After appropriate periods of incubating, the embryos were examined microscopically to identify their stages of development using the criteria developed by Hamburger and Hamilton (1951). Perfusion-fixation of the hearts were accomplished by injecting 3% glutaraldehyde in Tyrode's solution into a cannula that has been inserted in situ into a major vein. The hearts were then sectioned at one of 3

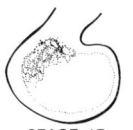
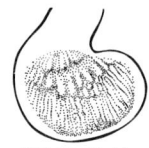
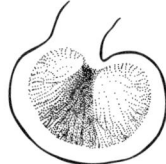
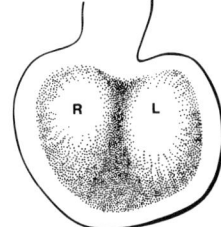

Figure 1
Schematic diagram of the primitive ventricular tube of the chick heart in the frontal projection, at incremental Hamburger-Hamilton stages of development. (A) At stage 17, early trabeculae formation is occurring in the bulboventricular region. (B) At stage 18-19, extensive trabeculations are present throughout the primitive ventricle. (C) At stage 26, there is increased concentration and early coalescence of the trabecular sheets at the cranial portion of the proximal ventricular loop. The caudal trabecular sheets are still unfused and relatively wide apart. (D) At stages 28-30, fusion of the trabecular sheets has continued further to include the caudal segments, resulting in completion of the formation of the muscular interventricular septum.

planes: coronal (frontal), transverse (horizontal), or sagittal (antero-posterior). The cut specimens were subjected to further fixation with glutaraldehyde, then staining with 1% osmium tetroxide, dehydration in alcohol and, finally, critical point drying. Following gold sputtering, the dehydrated specimens were examined with a scanning electron microscope, and were photographed. The technical details are reported elsewhere (Ben Schachar, Arcilla, Lucas, Manasek, 1985).

A summary of the structural changes within the cavity of the developing ventricle will now be presented. Changes in the size and shape of the ventricle, although mutually related to those of the intracavitary events, will not be discussed. They are presented in a more comprehensive report (Ben Schachar, Arcilla, Lucas, Manasek, 1985).

At stage 16 (age, 51-56 hours), the primitive ventricular tube (PVT) is still untrabeculated. Its inner surface is smooth and lined by endothelial cells. At its proximal end lies the common atrioventricular canal, and at its distal end is the bulbus cordis which continues into the truncus arteriosus.

At stage 17 (age 52-64 hours), the inner surface of the bulbar region and adjoining distal part of the PVT is now irregular due to beginning trabecular formation "Fig. 1A". The trabeculae consist of bundles of myocytes lined by endocardial cells. The rest of the PVT is still smooth-surfaced.

By stage 18-19 (age, 3-3½ days), there is abundant trabeculae throughout the PVT distributed more or less homogenously "Fig. 1B". They form trabecular bundles that are directed dorso-ventrally towards the floor of the PVT as well as towards its dorsal and ventral walls. These bundles become confluent by stage 20-22, forming lattice-like trabecular sheets of tissue that run also in dorso-ventral fashion. By this time, the ventricular loop is more acutely bent, forming in the process an angle that demarcates the proximal loop from the distal loop. The angle or groove between the two loops corresponds to an area inside the PVT which reveal increased concentration of the major trabecular bundles. Neither on coronal nor on transverse sections can a solid muscular septum be identified "Fig. 2".

At stage 23-26 (age 4-5 days), the trabecular sheets continue to be crowded and more concentrated at the cranial end of the proximal ventricular loop resulting in a flat trabecular plate of tissue. The caudal ends of the trabecular sheets are still wide apart, running dorso-ventrally in the proximal ventricular loop and in a somewhat circular manner in the distal ventricular loop. By stage 26, beginning coalescence of the dense cranial ends of the trabecular plates is observed, representing the initial process of septal formation "Fig. 3". As in the preceding stages, there is no identifiable solid muscular structure at the floor of the ventricle.

By stages 28-30 (age, 5½ to 7 days), there is continued fusion of the trabecular sheets not only at their cranial ends but, subsequently, at their distal ends also. This results in the formation of a thin muscular septum whose cranial crest becomes continuous with the superior septum originating from the atrioventricular endocardial cushions. The PVT is, by now, partitioned into two separate ventricles. From stage 30 on, further development of the muscular ventricular septum consists of progressive thickening due to continued coalescence of the adjoining trabecular sheets. The rest of the trabeculae become gradually plastered to the free walls of both ventricles which are also rapidly enlarging at this time.

Our study has thus demonstrated that the muscular ventricular septum develops through coalescence of trabeculae rather than through ventricular free wall outpocketing. The trabecular fusion starts cranially at the bulbo-ventricular area by around stage 26 and is more or less completed by stage 30. This results in a

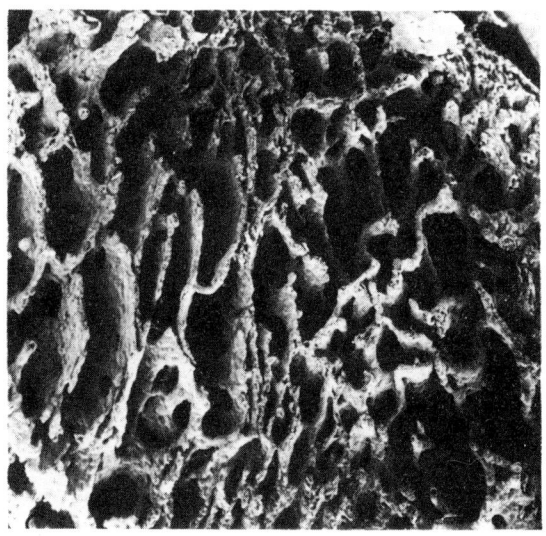

Figure 2
    Transverse section of primitive ventricular tube at caudal level close to its floor at stage 22, showing extensive trabecular sheets throughout and absence of a solid muscular structure. Magnification x 80.

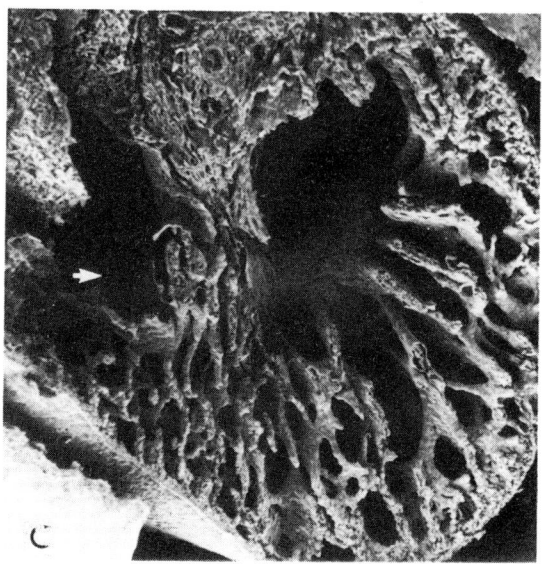

Figure 3
    Coronal section of primitive ventricle at stage 26, ventral view, showing coalesced trabecular sheets at cranial region but still unfused and well-separated trabecular sheets at caudal region towards the floor of the ventricle. Magnification x130. Cavity on left (white arrow) is in distal loop and belongs to future right ventricle; that on opposite side is in proximal loop and belongs to future left ventricle.

muscular septum that divides the primitive ventricle into separate right and left ventricles. A solid muscular structure at the floor of the primitive ventricle, serving as a precursor for the muscular ventricular septum, was not identified.

II. Intracardiac flow streaming
Microangiography consisting of injecting methylene blue solution into the peripheral veins of chick embryos was carried out in ovo. Our objective was to determine the flow patterns of the bloodstreams within the developing heart prior to septation and valve formation. The material consisted of 134 embryos in their early stages of development. These consisted of 15 embryos at H-H stage 14, 20 embryos at stages 15-16, 49 embryos at stages 17-18, and 50 embryos at stages 19-22. After appropriate incubation, the embryos were exposed by creating a window in the shell of the egg at its blunt end. The stage of development of each embryo was determined (Hamburger, Hamilton, 1951), and methylene blue microangiography (MBM) was then carried out.

MBM was performed under microscopy, using a glass micropipette whose tip varied from 1 to 6 μm in diameter, filled with 0.4% methylene blue solution. With the aid of a micromanipulator, the pipette was inserted at intervals into the following vitelline veins: 3 tributaries of the left lateral vitelline vein, 3 tributaries of the right lateral vitelline vein, left and right anterior vitelline veins, and left posterior vitelline vein. At each site, approximately 0.003-0.03 μl of the dye solution was slowly injected over a period of 2-5 seconds. The dye-containing venous stream was then followed visually under the microscope as it coursed through the omphalomesenteric trunk, heart, branchial arches and aorta, and was photographed. Most of the MBM studies were performed with the embryo lying in its usual position with its right side up on the yolk, i.e., in a right lateral position. In some, MBM was performed after gently turning the embryo into the opposite position, i.e., into a left lateral position. The technical details have been reported elsewhere (Yoshida, Manasek, Arcilla, 1983).

Bloodflow within the primary heart tube appeared to be laminar, enabling identification of the dye-containing and non-dye containing streams at any time "Figs. 4 and 5". As in previous reports, two intracardiac streams were also recognized. However, their course and orientation differed from those of Bremer and others (Bremer, 1932; Jafee, 1962; Jafee, 1965) who described a right heart stream and a left heart stream both of which assumed a spiral course at the conotruncus region. One stream (Type A), shown schematically by the dotted line in "Fig. 6", coursed along the dorsal wall of the common omphalomesenteric trunk and sinus venosus, proceeded to the cranial portion of the primitive atrium and atrioventricular canal, and then coursed into the ventral portion of the primitive ventricle and conus cordis. It then turned clockwise about 90° toward the aortic arches, reaching preferentially the left branchial arches. The other stream (Type B), illustrated by the solid line, ran along the ventral wall of the common omphalomesenteric trunk and sinus venosus, proceeded to the caudal region of the primitive atrium and atrioventricular canal, and then coursed into the dorsal portion of the primitive ventricle and conus cordis, before finally rotating for about 90° to preferentially reach the right branchial arches. Thus, both streams maintained cranio-caudal relations within the primitive atrium but antero-posterior relations within the primitive ventricle and conus cordis.

Flow streaming in the branchial arches and in the dorsal aorta was most unusual. Type A stream continued preferentially into the left arches whereas Type B stream chiefly continued into the right arches. In addition, streaming of flow was notable in the dorsal aorta to the extent that the Type A stream continued mostly into the left vitelline artery and its branches whereas the Type B stream continued preferentially into the right vitelline artery and its branches "Fig. 7".

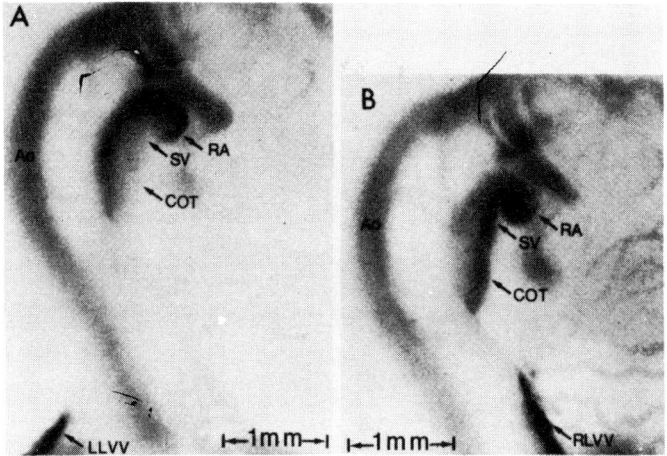

Figure 4
Microangiograms in chick embryos at H-H stage 19. (A) showing Type A stream after methylene blue injection into left lateral vitelline vein (LLVV). Note dorsal distribution of dye stream in common omphalomesenteric trunk (COT) and sinus venosus (SV), and cranial orientation in the primitive atrium (RA). (B) Showing Type B stream after dye injection into right lateral vitelline vein (RLVV). Note ventral distribution of dye stream in the omphalomesenteric trunk and sinus venosus, and caudal distribution in primitive atrium. Reprinted from Circ Res 53:363, 1983.

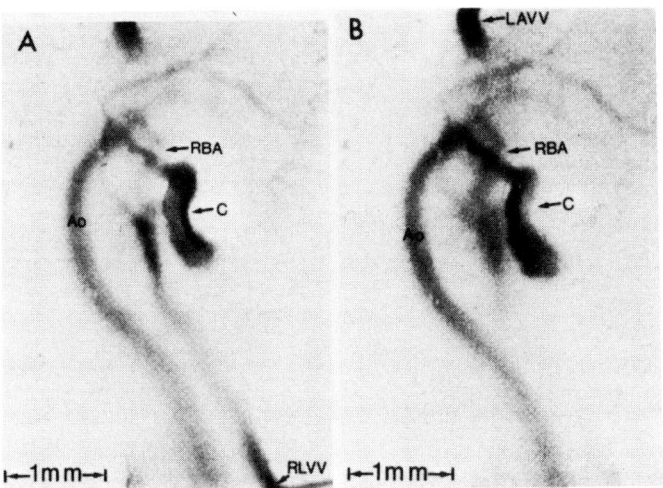

Figure 5
Microangiograms at H-H stage 17. (A) Showing Type A stream after methylene blue injection into right lateral vitelline vein (RLVV), with anterior orientation in primitive ventricle and conus cordis (C). (B) Showing Type B stream after dye injection into left anterior vitelline vein (LAVV), with posterior orientation in primitive ventricle and conus. Reprinted from Circ Res 53:363, 1983.

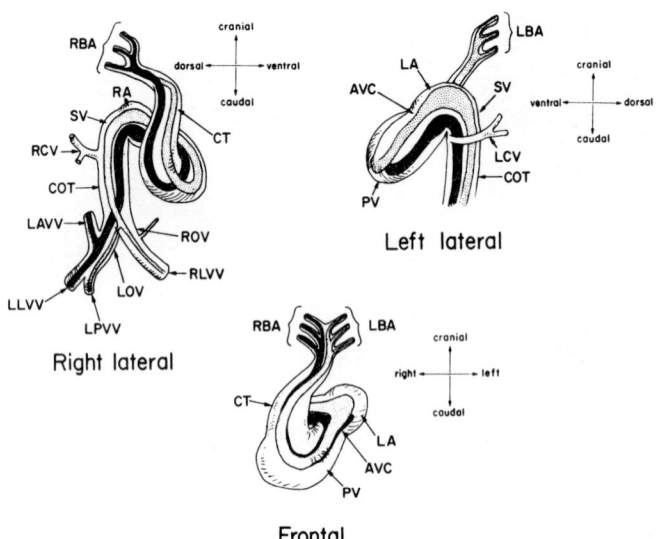

Figure 6
    Diagram of the Type A stream (dotted) and of the Type B stream (solid) within the primary heart tube as viewed in the frontal, right lateral and left lateral projections. RA - right side of primitive atrium, LA - left side of primitive atrium, AVC - atrioventricular canal, PV - primitive ventricle, CT - conotruncus, RBA - right branchial arches, LBA - left branchial arches. Reprinted from Circ Res 53:363, 1983.

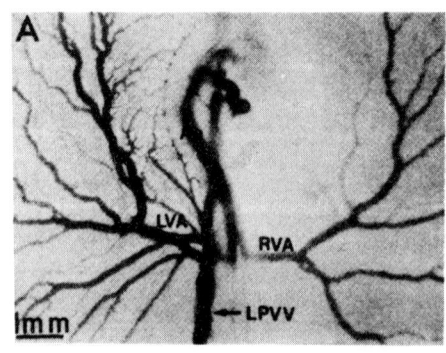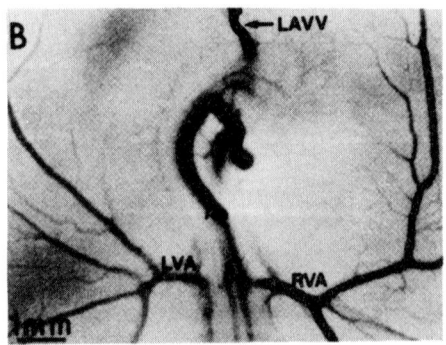

Figure 7
    Microangiograms at H-H stages 15-16, demonstrating unusual streaming of flow along dorsal aorta. (A) Type A stream originating from left posterior vitelline vein (LPVV) selectively flowing into the left vitelline artery (LVA) and branches. (B) Type B stream from left anterior vitelline vein (LAVV) which selectively flows into the right vitelline artery (RVA) and branches. Reprinted from Circ Res 53:363, 1983.

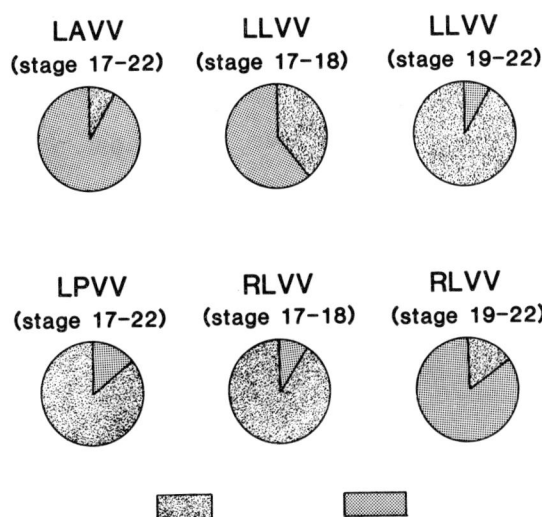

Figure 8 Streaming patterns of peripheral venous returns at various stages of development. Frequency of intracardiac streaming pattern is given in percent. Note shift of streaming patterns by the lateral vitelline veins between H-H stages 17-18 and H-H stages 19-22. LAVV - left anterior vitelline vein, LPVV - left posterior vitelline vein, LLVV - left lateral vitelline vein, RLVV - right lateral vitelline vein.

The unusual orientation of the two intracardiac streams, demonstrated in this study, does not fully support the flow-molding theory which suggests that the streaming of flow within the developing heart promotes septation at the ventricular, bulbar and truncal levels. The cranio-caudal relations of the two streams within the primitive atrium and common atrioventricular canal cannot account for the eventual right-left and antero-posterior relations of the right and left atria in the fully-developed heart. By the same token, the strictly antero-posterior relations of the streams within the proximal and distal ventricular loops, including conus cordis, fails to account for the specific orientation of the fully-developed interventricular septum and the relative positions of the right and left ventricles. Since the streams at the conotruncus do not follow a spiral course, at least during the early stages of cardiac development, the likelihood that these streams play a major role in conotruncal septation is also not too convincing. Finally, the unusual streaming pattern in the branchial arches and aorta is such that if the conotruncal septum was to follow the direction of the two streams along these vessels, each ventricle would end up selectively perfusing half of the body through its own set of arteries. Our observations instead support the concept that septation, just like other basic developmental events, appears to be intrinsic or programmed.

Since the injection sites were the same in virtually all the embryos studied, the venous origins of the Type A and Type B streams were identified (Yoshida, Manasek, Arcilla, 1983). Generally speaking, the left posterior vitelline vein contributed to the Type A stream whereas the left anterior vitelline vein continued as the Type B stream. At H-H stages 17-18, venous return from the right lateral vitelline vein and from the left lateral vitelline vein continued as Type A and Type B streams, respectively. At H-H stages 19-22, venous return from these veins was the reverse. By now, the right lateral vitelline vein chiefly continued as Type B stream whereas the left lateral vitelline vein preferentially continued as Type A stream "Fig. 8". This information relative to the venous components of each intracardiac stream, at incremental stages of embryonic development, is essential to future experimental studies dealing with perturbation of venous flow in the developing embryo and its effects upon cardiac development.

ACKNOWLEDGEMENT

I gratefully acknowledge the invaluable assistance of a few colleagues without whom this work would not have been possible. Dr. Giora Ben Schachar (currently, Assistant Professor of Pediatrics, Case Western Reserve University, Cleveland) was responsible for study #1 on the development of muscular interventricular septum, Dr. Hitoshi Yoshida (currently, Associate Professor of Pediatrics, Kanazawa University, Kanazawa, Japan) was responsible for study #2 on intracardiac flow streaming. Dr. Frank Manasek, Associate Professor of Anatomy and Pediatrics, The University of Chicago, unselfishly provided guidance, ideas and constant encouragement. I also acknowledge, with great fondness, the help and guidance of John Lind during my early scientific career and his unfailing friendship through the years. To his memory, I dedicate this paper.

REFERENCES

Ben Schachar, G., Arcilla, R.A., Lucas, R.V., Manasek, F.J. (1985): Ventricular trabeculations in the chick embryo heart and their contribution to ventricular and muscular septal development. In Press

Bremer, J.L. (1932): The presence and influence of two spiral streams in the heart of the chick embryo. Am J Anat 49:409-440.

Chang, C. (1932): On the reaction of the endocardium to the blood stream in the embryonic heart with special reference to the endocardial thickenings in the atrioventricular canal and bulbous cordis. Anat Rec 51:253-265.

Hamburger, V., Hamilton, H.L. (1951): A series of normal stages in the development of the chick embryo. J Morphol 88:49-92.

Hibbs, R.V. (1956): Electron microscopy of developing cardiac muscle in chick embryos. Am J Anat 99:17-51.

Jafee, O.C. (1962): Hemodynamics and cardiogenesis. The effects of altered vascular patterns on cardiac development. J Morphol 110:217-225.

Jafee, O.C. (1965): Hemodynamic factors in the development of the chick embryo heart. Anat Rec 151:69-76.

Manasek, F.J. (1968): Embryonic development of the heart. I. A light and electron microscopic study of myocardial development in the early chick embryo. J Morphol 125:329-365.

Morse, D.E. (1978): Scanning electron microscopy of the developing septa in the chick heart. In Morphogenesis and Malformation of the Cardiovascular System. The National Foundation March of Dimes, Birth Defects Original Article Series Vol. XIV, No 7, pp 91-107, Rosenquist G.C. and Bergsma D., ed, Alan R. Liss, New York.

Patten, B.M., Kramer, T.C. (1933): The initiation of contraction in the embryonic chick heart. Am J Anat 53:349-375.

Patten, B.M. (1951): Development of the chick during the third and fourth days of incubation. In Early Embryology of the Chick, McGraw-Hill Inc., New York, pp 156-213.

Streeter, G.L. (1948): Developmental Horizons in Human Embryos. Description of Age Groups XV, XVI, XVII, and XVIII. Carnegie Contrib Embryol 32:133-203.

Yoshida, H., Manasek, F.J., Arcilla, R.A. (1983): Intracardiac flow patterns in early embryonic life. A reexamination. Circ Res 53:363-371.

Supported in part by: NIH Grant No. HL-13831.

RESUME

Le rôle des courants sanguins intra-cardiaques dans la morphogénèse cardiaque et la septation bulbo-ventriculaire a été étudié sur des embryons de poulets (coeur facilement accessible, stdes de développement identifiables avec précision selon les descriptions de Hamburger et Hamilton, 1951: stades H-H.)

Les premières contractions cardiaques sont visibles au stade H-H 10, au moment de l'inflexion en boucle du tube cardiaque primitif. La circulation sanguine débute au stade 12. Le cloisonnement cardiaque est beaucoup plus tardif (commençant au niveau auriculaire vers le stade 16-17 et au niveau ventriculaire vers le stade 26). Durant la période où la circulation sanguine est entretenue par un coeur à 2 cavités sans valves, des courants droit et gauche ont été vus en observation directe; d'autre part, les travaux antérieurs basés sur des reconstructions et sur l'histologie n'ont pas réglé le problème de la morphogénèse du septum interventriculaire. Ces points ont donc été repris dans les deux études présentées ici, effectuées avec des techniques récentes beaucoup plus sophistiquées.

1) Le développement du septum interventriculaire a été analysé par microscopie électronique, sur 62 coeurs embryonnaires étagés du stade

H-H 16 au stade 39 (détails techniques, voir Ben Schachar et al., 1985). Au stade 16, le tube ventriculaire primitif (TVP) est encore lisse; la trabéculation apparait à l'extrémité distale du TVP et au niveau du bulbe au stade 17, et elle forme des faisceaux abondants aux stades 18-19. Ces faisceux confluent et s'entrelacent en réseaux, formant des feuillets qui se mettent en place dans le sens dorso-ventral aux stades 20-22. A ce moment, la boucle cardiaque serrée détermine une angulation marquée entre la zone proximale et la zone distale du TVP, à laquelle correspond, à l'intérieur du TVP, une concentration marquée de trabéculations. Aux stades 26-30, les feuillets deviennent coalescents, <u>d'abord dans la région bulbo-ventriculaire</u>, en s'étendant vers le plancher du TVP pour former le septum interventriculaire musculaire. Le reste des trabéculations va progressivement s'attacher aux parois externes des ventricules dont le volume croît rapidement.

2) Les courants intra-cardiaques ont été étudiés par microangiographie au bleu de méthylène, en injectant <u>in ovo</u> 9 veines vitellines périphériques, sur 134 embryons étagés du stade H-H 14 au stade 22 (sous microscope et avec un micromanipulateur, détails techniques voir Yoshida et al., 1983). Deux types de courants intra-cardiaques ont été identifiés et photographiés: le courant type A longe le segment cranial de l'oreillette primitive et du canal atrio-ventriculaire (AV), puis il suit la région ventrale du TVP et du bulbe, se dirigeant alors préférentiellement vers les arcs branchiaux gauches Le courant de type B côtoie les zones caudales de l'oreillette primitive et du canal AV, puis serre la région dorsale du TVP et du bulbe, et se dirige plutôt vers les arcs branchiaux droits. Les deux courant restent parallèles en traversant le TVP, et ne se tordent nullement en spirale. La persistance des courants A et B dans l'aorte dorsale est remarquable, et elle se maintient jusqu'à l'origine des artères vitellines (figure 7).

Ces résultats ne sont pas en faveur de la théorie selon laquelle la morphogénèse cardiaque serait façonnée par les courants sanguins ("flow-molding"), mais ils donnent à penser que le développement cardiaque précoce suit une ligne intrinsèque ou programmée.

****

DISCUSSION. Dr. L. Stern moderator.

<u>Dr. W. Oh</u>: Was timing of the experiments in the traditional studies by previous investigators the same to your own studies?

<u>Dr. R. Arcilla</u>: No. The earlier studies were, as I have briefly mentioned, based primarily on the forwards movements of the red cells within and outside the embryonic heart. From our experience, it is virtually impossible to determine the precise orientations of the two intracardiac streams in their entirety as contrasted, for example, with the methylene blue injection technic. Many of the earlier studies were also carried out at comparatively later stges of development whereas we have specifically done ours before septal development has occurred. So it is possible that the two observations (namely that by Bremer and other earlier investigators and our own investigations) are not necessarily contradictory. It is necessary, however, that we extend our microangiography study to older embryos to clarify this point.

Dr. B. Lundell: Would you say that there is a similar intrinsic programming also for the formation and growth of the valves and great arteries and not only for the myocardial structures?

Dr. R. Arcilla: Yes, I strongly suspect that the very early stages of cardio-vascular development are intrinsically programmed. As a matter of fact, this is probably true for all developing systems as well. There is no doubt, for example, that cell differentiation and growth is for the most part intrinsic although embryonic environmental factors may influence cell size and number later on, as is the case with the myocardial cells exposed to fetal cardiac overload. I also believe that the formation of the cardiac valvular structures, of the arterial tree and of the primitive veins is a similarly programmed phenomenon although also subject to circulatory changes at later stages of development, comparatively speaking, based on hydrodynamic principles.

Dr. J. Warshaw: Is this programming seen in culture? Does the *in vitro* situation mirror what is going on *in vivo*?

Dr. R. Arcilla: The organ culture technic has been used to analyze certain processes of cardiac development. In one study that I am aware of, for example, Manasek (Dev Biol 1972, *27*:584) has shown that spontaneous looping of the chick primary heart tube that is growing in culture still occurs despite total depression of cardiac contractions by high potassium in the culture media. This study provides convincing evidence for intrinsic programming independent of cardiac function. We are also currently utilizing organ culture technics to determine the influence of venous perturbation, now that the venous components of the intracardiac streams have been identified, upon the venous circulation, intracardiac streaming and cardiac development using our chick embryo model.

Fetal echocardiography and Doppler blood flow studies

D.M. Friedman

Pediatric Cardiology, New York University Medical Center, 550 First Avenue, New York, NY 10016, USA

ABSTRACT

Fetal echocardiography is becoming widely available, and we are seeing an increasing use of M-mode and two-dimensional, real-time imaging techniques, as well as Doppler blood velocity recordings. These techniques are particularly appropriate for use in high-risk groups, which include cases of intrauterine growth retardation and fetal dysrhythmias, as well as polyhydramnios and suspected non-immune fetal hydrops. Maternal heart disease, drug exposures, diabetes, hypertension, collagen vascular disease, RH sensitization, or family histories of congenital heart disease are further indications for fetal echocardiography.

This analysis may be used to assess fetal growth parameters, such as estimations of gestational age, or the presence of growth retardation. One is able to explore the developmental patterns of normal prenatal circulation. Fetal echocardiography is useful in making specific diagnoses of congenital heart disease, and for analyzing fetal dysrhythmias. The analysis of fetal well-being is available by determining the degree of non-immune fetal hydrops. More recently, Doppler blood velocity wave form analysis in the umbilical vessels are used in assessing fetal well-being.

KEY WORDS

Fetal echocardiography
Fetal Doppler

I. INTRODUCTION

Fetal cardiac ultrasound has evolved over the past decade to include M-mode, two-dimensional and Doppler technology. This technique is informative, reproducible, serially applicable, economical, and readily available. Of note is the non-invasive nature and safety of the method for the fetus (Baker and Dalrymple, 1978; Scheidt et al, 1978). Fetal echocardiography provides information on structure, growth, and function of the developing cardiovascular system.

II. PATIENT SELECTION AND TIMING

Although fetal cardiac structures may be visualized as early as 16 to 18 weeks of gestation, elective cases provide technically optimal studies at 28 to 34 weeks. Examinations are generally restricted to high-risk groups, including intrauterine growth retardation and fetal dysrhythmias, as well as polyhydramnios and suspected non-immune fetal hydrops, a form of in utero congestive heart failure. Other factors included in this group are maternal heart disease, drug exposures, diabetes, hypertension, collagen vascular disease, Rh sensitization, or family histories of congenital heart disease.

III. INDICATIONS AND USES

Cardiac ultrasound can evaluate fetal growth parameters, such as estimations of gestational age, or the presence of growth retardation. Normal developmental patterns of prenatal circulation can be directly assessed non-invasively. The recognition of many forms of congenital heart disease is now possible prenatally, as well as the analysis of fetal dysrhythmias. The concept of fetal well-being is evaluated by the degree of non-immune fetal hydrops, as well as in the analysis of Doppler blood velocity waveforms in the umbilical vessels.

A. Developmental Anatomy

Sahn et al (1980) have had extensive experience with both qualitative and quantitative aspects of fetal echocardiography. A large, serial study of normal pregnancies using M-mode and two-dimensional echocardiographic techniques produced adequate visualization in over 90% of the cases, and established normal growth curves of fetal cardiac dimensions. When compared to estimated fetal weights, the correlations were strong. Furthermore, their data statistically demonstrated the presence of a prenatal right ventricular size predominance over the left ventricle, which was no longer present prenatally. This phenomenon was interpreted as being consistent with the predictions of hemodynamic conditions in utero as shown by Rudolph's studies (1974) on the fetal lamb model, which consist of a right ventricular volume overload pattern. Roczen's (1981) quantitative fetal M-mode echocardiographic study of normal pregnancies also confirmed a fetal right ventricular volume overload pattern consisting of predominently flat interventricular septal motion.

Conversely, Wladimiroff and McGhie (1981) were unable to confirm a right ventricular preponderance pattern in their normative study which quantitated M-mode and two-dimensional data in a large series of normal gestations. They pointed out, however, that controversy over the sheep data persists as well.

B. Congenital Anomalies

Kleinman et al (1980) have studied several hundred patients in specific high-risk groups, which include fetuses suspected of having congenital anomalies or arrhythmias, including intrauterine growth retardation. Maternal or familial risk factors such as the presence of heart disease, diabetes, hypertension, collagen vascular disease, or exposure to potential teratogens are indications for study. After extensive experience, they have diagnosed many specific forms of congenital heart disease or arrhythmias prenatally, and even offered some limited therapeutic options.

C. Fetal Arrhythmias and Transplacental Therapy

Fetal echocardiography, especially M-mode data, is useful in analyzing fetal arrhythmias. Kleinman et al (1983) have shown that most of these patients present with polyhydramnios and non-immune fetal hydrops, or with an auscultatory arrhythmia. The common types were supraventricular and self-limited, including atrial premature beats or sinus slowing. However, sustained fetal arrhythmias such as atrial flutter or tachycardia, or complete heart block, were often associated with structural heart disease, and carried a grave prognosis.

Transplacental therapy of fetal arrhythmias has occasionally been successful, such as supraventricular tachycardias treated with digoxin, propranolol, or procainamide (Dumesic et al, 1982). Early Cesarean section for refractory arrhythmias is an additional treatment option (Belhassen et al, 1982).

D. Non-Immune Fetal Hydrops

Congenital heart disease is a common cause of non-immune fetal hydrops, even in the absence of arrhythmias. Kleinman et al (1982) have diagnosed many forms of structural heart disease prenatally when examined for this indication. The earliest cases included transposition of the great vessels, tetralogy of Fallot, atrioventricular canal, ventricular septal defects, valvular lesions, cardiac tumors, myocardial infarctions, Ebstein's anomaly, and polysplenia syndrome.

E. Functional Status - The Concept of Fetal "Well-Being"

A tool for direct assessment of the dynamic functional status of the fetal circulation would be invaluable to both the clinician and researcher. Early attempts in this field included the Doppler and electrocardiographic measurement of prenatal systolic time intervals by Wolfson et al (1977), illustrating the progressive prolongation of pre-ejection period with advancing gestational age.

The development of Doppler techniques to directly measure fetal blood flows has produced exciting new information. Stuart et al (1980) analyzed serial Doppler blood velocity waveforms from the umbilical artery in normal pregnancies. These characteristic waveforms consist of a maximal systolic blood velocity, point A, and a least diastolic velocity, point B, as well as their ratio, A/B. A systemic, predictable increase in the diastolic blood flow in the umbilical artery occurs with advancing gestational age, presumably reflecting the normal maturational fall in placental vascular resistance. No significant changes in these hemodynamic characteristics occurred during normal labor and its interventions (Stuart et al, 1981). It would be predicted, however, that an abnormal elevation of placental vascular resistance, such as the result of placental pathology, might result in a lessening of forward diastolic flow in the umbilical artery, manifested as an elevated A/B ratio.

Giles et al (1982) also analyzed the A/B ratio in the umbilical artery Doppler blood velocity waveforms, confirming the normal decrease with advancing gestational age. Strikingly, they demonstrated the ability of the A/B ratio to predict the loss of fetal well-being in a large population of high-risk pregnancies. Of 44 abnormal values, 37 gestations resulted in intrauterine growth retardation, stillbirths, or fetal distress. Such predictions of the loss of fetal well-being by a decrease in the diastolic velocity of Doppler umbilical artery waveforms were confirmed by McCallum et al (1978).

F. Measurement of Blood Flow

Doppler measurements of fetal and neonatal blood flows have confirmed some of the findings for humans extrapolated from animal studies. Reid et al (1980) found excellent agreement between their Doppler data and the classic values published in the literature from invasive animal studies for fetal blood flows. Gill (1979, 1981) measured prenatal umbilical venous flow from Doppler blood velocity techniques. The quantitative umbilical venous return represents the effective fetal cardiac output. This value is normally remarkably constant per unit of body weight with advancing gestational age, thus potentially providing another index of gestational age or fetal well-being.

IV. SUMMARY

Advanced techniques in fetal echocardiography, including Doppler blood velocity measurements, are now widely available, allowing the non-invasive assessment of gestational age, fetal growth patterns, cardiac anatomy and function, as well as an indication of fetal well-being. The techniques should be restricted to high-risk groups suspected of arrhythmias, congenital anomalies, or fetal distress.

Should a positive examination be found, various options are presently available. Transplacental drug therapy has been effective, as well as planned early delivery. Alerting the perinatal staff and family in order to plan in advance for anticipated problems is of obvious benefit. Multiple congenital anomalies can be assessed, as well as serial evaluations of circulatory status. Under certain circumstances, early abortion may be elected.

Various aspects of this field are still preliminary, but it promises exciting advances in the near future.

REFERENCES

Baker, M.L. and Dalrymple, G.V. (1978): Biological effects of diagnostic ultrasound: A review. Radiology 126, 479-483.

Belhassen, B., Pauzner, D., Blieden, L., Sherez, J., Zinger, A., David, M., Muhlbauer, B., and Laniado, S. (1982): Intrauterine and postnatal atrial fibrillation in the Wolff-Parkinson-White syndrome. Circulation 66, 1124-1128.

Dumesic, D.H., Silverman, N.H., Tobias, S., and Golbus, M.S. (1982): Transplacental cardioversion of fetal supraventricular tachycardia with procainamide. New Engl. J. Med. 307, 1128-1131.

Giles, W.B., Trudinger, B.J., and Cook, C.M. (1982): Fetal umbilical artery velocity waveforms. J. Ultrasound Med. 1 (Suppl.), 98.

Gill, R.W. (1979): Pulsed Doppler with B-mode imaging for quantitative blood flow measurement. Prog. Med. Biol. 5, 223-235.

Gill, G.W. Trudinger, B.J. Garrett, W.J., Kossoff, G., and Warren, P.S. (1981): Fetal umbilical venous flow measured in utero by pulsed Doppler and B-mode ultrasound. Am. J. Obstet. Gynecol. 139, 720-725.

Kleinman, C.S., Hobbins, J.C., Jaffe, C.C., Lynch, D.C., and Talner, N.S. (1980): Echocardiographic studies of the human fetus: Prenatal diagnosis of congenital heart disease and cardiac dysrhythmias. Pediatrics 65, 1059-1067.

Kleinman, C.S., Donnerstein, R.L., DeVore, G.R., Jaffe, C.C., Lynch, D.C., Berkowitz, R.L., Talner, N.S., and Hobbins, J.C. (1982): Fetal echocardiography for evaluation of in utero congestive heart failure. New Engl. J. Med. 306, 568-574.

Kleinman, C.S., Donnerstein, R.L., Jaffe, C.C., DeVore, G.R., Weinstein, E.M., Lynch, D.C., Talner, N.S., Berkowitz, R.L., and Hobbins, J.C. (1983): Fetal echocardiography. Am. J. Cardiol. 51, 237-243.

McCallum, W.D., Williams, C.S., Napel, S., and Daigle, R.E. (1978): Fetal blood velocity waveforms. Am. J. Obstet Gynecol. 132, 425-429.

Reid, M.H. Mackay, R.S., and Lantz, B.M.T. (1980): Non-invasive measurement of fetal and neonatal blood flow. Acta Radiol. [Diagn.] 21, 197-202.

Roczen, R.S. (1981): Fetal echocardiography: Present and future applications. J. Clin. Ultrasound 9, 223-229.

Rudolph, A.M. (1974): Congenital Diseases of the Heart. Yearbook Medical Publishers, Chicago, pp. 1-16.

Sahn, D.J., Lange, L.W., Allen, H.D., Goldberg, S.J., Anderson, C., Giles, H., and Haber, K. (1980): Quantitative real-time cross-sectional echocardiography in the developing normal human fetus and newborn. Circulation 62, 588-597.

Scheidt, P.C., Stanley, F., and Bryla, D.A. (1978): One-year follow-up of infants exposed to ultrasound in utero. Am. J. Obstet. Gynecol. 131, 743-748.

Stuart, B., Drumm, J., Fitzgerald, D.E., and Duigan, N.M. (1980). Fetal blood velocity waveforms in normal pregnancy. Br. J. Obstet. Gynaecol. 87, 780-785.

Stuart, B., Drumm, J., Fitzgerald, D.E., and Duigan, N.M. (1981): Fetal blood velocity waveforms in uncomplicated labour. Br. J. Obstet. Gynaecol. 88, 865-869.

Wladimiroff, J.W. and McGhie, J.S. (1981): M-mode ultrasonic assessment of fetal cardiovascular dynamics. Br. J. Obstet. Gynaecol. 88, 1241-1245.

Wolfson, R.N., Zador, I.E., Pillay, S.K. Timor-Tritsch, I.E., and Hertz, R.H. (1977): Antenatal investigation of human fetal systolic time intervals. Am. J. Obstet. Gynecol. 129, 203-207.

RESUME.

Au cours de la dernière décennie, l'échocardiographie foetale s'est enrichie des techniques en M-mode, en imagerie bi-dimensionnelle en temps réel, et en enregistrement Doppler des vélocités du flux sanguin. Elle fournit maintenant des informations sur les structures cardiaques, leur croissance, et l'aspect fonctionnel du système cardio-vasculaire en cours de développement. Les meilleures visualisations sont obtenues entre 28 et 34 semaines, mais parfois des images suffisantes peuvent être obtenues dès 16-18 semaines. Les indications se limitent aux groupes de mères à haut risque: cardiopathie chez la mère ou dans la famille, dysrythmies foetales, retards de croissance intra-utérins, polyhydramnios, anasarque sans incompatibilité Rhesus, diabète ou hypertension ou maladie du collagène chez la mère. En dehors du diagnostic maintenant classique des cardiopathies congénitales et/ou des arythmies foetales, l'utilisation des techniques Doppler pour l'estimation des débits sanguins foetaux a permis de prédire une altération de l'état foetal au vu de la diminution de la composante diastolique du débit dans l'artère ombilicale. Quand l'échocardiographie foetale relève une anomalie, diverses attitudes sont possibles: traiter une arythmie par voie transplacentaire (digoxine, propanolol), avancer la date de l'accouchement, alerter la famille et l'équipe périnatale pour préparer un accueil approprié au nouveau-né atteint, enfin recourir à l'interruption de grossesse dans certains cas particuliers.

****

DISCUSSION. Dr.L.STERN, moderator.

Dr L Stern: What new ethical issues have arisen? We already had enough troubles with the old ones...

Dr.D.Friedman: Some workers, for instance, have diagnosed hypoplastic left heart syndrome, a virtually universally fatal lesion, at 18-20 weeks of gestation (N.Silverman, J.Amer.Coll.Cardiol.1985; 5:20S-29S). Under such circumstances, depending upon the family's wishes and one's current management options, referral for therapeutic abortion might be considered.

Dr.B.Lundell: We can accept a rather low sensitivity when a new technique is introduced, but if we intend to give advice on abortion based on our findings, the specificity must be very close to 100%. What is the current accuracy of this technique in predicting a severe morbidity or high mortality after birth in a heart malformation?

Dr.D.Friedman: I cannot comment on this matter from my own data. However, a recent review by Drs.N.Silverman and M.Golbus (J.Amer.Coll. Cardiol. 1985; 5:20S-29S) discusses this uncertainty, stating:"Since the acquisition of the latest equipment...we made no major errors.... It is remarkable that even with the potential for error...the technique has been precise, as attested to by the extensive list of confirmed abnormalities that have been recognized". Dr.Ch.Kleinman has also been able to successfully image fetal hearts in 95% of cases between 18 and 40 weeks of gestation (J.Amer.Coll.Cardiol.1985; 5:84S-94S). In addition, each center will have its own learning curve, but I expect that sensitivities and specificities near 80 to 90% should be anticipated for most major lesions.

Dr.L.Stern: As long as all you want to do is prepare people for what may or may not occur, you do not have to worry whether you are at 89% or less. If you are going to interrupt a pregnancy on the basis of what you find, you had better get to 100% or as close as possible to it!

Dr.Ab.Rudolph: With some lesions, there is almost absolute specificity and accuracy. Some lesions, such as ventricular septal defect, may not be detected with as high a level of accuracy. However, I have been impressed with the accuracy of the more major and more severe anomalies.

Dr.W.Oh: Isn't it critical to know when to screen what?

Dr.D.Friedman: We start screening at 18 weeks in our high-risk cases, especially in women referred from the genetic clinic for previous personal or family history of congenital heart disease (CHD), or at any time when an arrhythmia is heard. If we get good visualization at 18 weeks, that is marvelous. If we don't, then we can recall these women in a week or so. Fetal echocardiography is not necessarily a tachnique which can be done in every case quickly in a 20-minute examination. One is relying here not on a fixed echo window. Rather, the fetus is moving in utero so that changes in fetal position may entirely change the success of an examination. Therefore, we begin our serial studies at 18 weeks.

Dr.J.Warshaw: Even in your highest risk group, how cost-effective is your screening?

Dr.D.Friedman: I don't have any figures at all on cost effectiveness of such a technique. I can tell you from personal experience that obtaining a normal fetal echocardiogram in a mother who is paricularly worried about her third or fourth pregnancy, following several children with CHD, is very reassuring.

Dr. L. Stern: But there are many different types of hereditary CHD that you deal with, so that the issue of cost effectiveness becomes a problem not only in terms of money but also in terms of time, even for the most efficient echocardiographer. Can you eliminate a certain number of candidates whose abnormalities are diagnosable by other means? I think the issue here is how early are you going to screen and how are you going to select the patients? You don't want to do everybody at 18 weeks.

Dr. D. Friedman: The obstetricians at this point are restricting the studies only to those selected high-risk groups I have mentioned. So far, the number of studies is still manageable.

Dr. Ab. Rudolph: I would like to raise an important issue relating to species differences. Several investigators using ultrasound assessment of fetal ventricular output in humans have attempted to relate left and right ventricular output to the measurements we have reported in fetal lambs. However, there is no reason to believe that right ventricular output should be double that of the left ventricle in the human fetus. The left ventricle provides blood to the brain and heart, as well as to the upper body. The fetal lamb has a brain weight equivalent to about 3 per cent of body weight, whereas the human fetal brain is about 13 per cent of body weight. Obviously, left ventricular output would be considerably higher in the human fetus than in the lamb. I have made some calculations assuming that brain blood flow per unit weight is similar in the lamb and human fetus, and have estimated that right ventricular output in the human fetus should be only about 1.2 times greater then left ventricular output. Recent studies of Doppler technique in human fetus tend to confirm this relationship.

Fetal–neonatal circulation revisited

S. Zoe Walsh

Norrtull's Hospital, Stockholm, Sweden.
(Correspondence: S.Z. Walsh, Ekshäradsgatan 87, 123 46 Farsta, Sweden)

ABSTRACT

I have tried here to review a few of the more salient changes in attitude towards the fetus. In this connection some of John Lind's contributions in the field of fetal and neonatal cardiovascular physiology have been mentioned - likewise the methodological aspects of the pediatric electrocardiogram. In addition, various studies are presented which throw light on the pattern of changes in the neonatal electrocardiogram.

Reminiscences about John Lind, pediatric ECG methods, ECG findings in newborns.

INTRODUCTION

At this symposium we are honoring the memory of John Lind. There are various ways of doing this, including the presentation of work in this area and sharing with you some recollections of the man himself. I have chosen a bit of both.

Abroad Johnny Lind was particularly well known for his work in the field of fetal and neonatal cardiovascular physiology. At home in Sweden he was regarded as a pioneer in all aspects of fetal and neonatal research. Not only did he participate in and support many research projects dealing with this age group but he took an active part in discussions and gave lectures and talks to the general public at meetings and in radio and television programs. Some of his favorite topics concerned rooming-in, active participation by fathers in the care of their infants and children (which he knew something about as the father of four), play therapy, and the importance of music for the fetus and newborn. Thus Johnny has many colleagues in Sweden who would have liked to be with us today.

When I went to work for Johnny in 1960, one of his first remarks was, "Well, I think you may find it hard to get used to life here. It may take a long while". He repeated this now and then. I know he thought the climate was difficult to get accustomed to and that first year it rained almost continuously. In the newspapers at that time I was surprised to read that in November 1960 there were four hours of sunshine and in December 85 minutes of sunshine. I missed it all.

In order to help me over any feelings of homesickness, Johnny placed me in a room beside his and would come for a chat several times each day. Occasionally he would hang up one of his paintings in my room in front of my desk and ask whether I liked it. Nearly always I didn´t like it for as I remember they were largely dark landscapes or very modern smears, stripes or dots. He changed it sometimes to cheer me up.

He had recently become Professor and Chairman of the Department of Pediatrics at Karolinska Hospital and Karolinska Institute, a post which entitled him to participate in the august group that selects Nobel Prize winners. He had a large staff of physicians, nurses, technicians and other personnel and a small group of foreign research workers, mainly from North America and Britain, most of whom were working on projects in the field of fetal and neonatal cardiovascular physiology. So the competition for babies for our respective studies was stiff at times, but always friendly. The weekly conference of the Pediatric Department was held in English for the benefit of the many visitors from abroad, as well as for the staff, since this was good practice for them if they wanted to present papers or work abroad.

When no deliveries were expected and he had visitors who were interested in our particular projects he would send us off together with some colleagues and staff to a museum. We would spend part of the time talking about our work and the rest taking in some culture and a meal at a museum where Johnny would come to join us. Thus he created a special atmosphere of comradeship which must be difficult to find in the average department of pediatrics today (Fig 1).

Johnny never told me a word about the beauty of Stockholm but often asked me what I thought of it. I always replied that Stockholm was lovely, that every day I discovered something new, and so on. Then he would merely nod. Two or three years later, a visitor came and Johnny asked her the same question. To my surprise her answer was, "It´s terrible. I used to like it but now it´s been ruined by the city planners. The place is all torn up. Now there are lots of cities in Europe which are prettier." Johnny showed no change of expression. Then he turned to me. "Zoe, what do you think of Stockholm?" He knew I would say that Stockholm was wonderful. And of course I said so. His face showed no change of expression then either, but he had hidden it with one hand.

Although Johnny Lind had a good sense of humor I cannot remenber hearing him tell a joke. I also cannot remember seeing him show a cartoon at a meeting. I suspect he would have felt uncomfortable doing so as he preferred to keep a low profile on such occasions don´t know whether he even liked cartoons but after we had decided to collaborate on a long chapter he gave me his office at Norrtull´s Hospital so that I could leave all the articles, books and figures spread out there. He sometimes brought people to see me and the mess as well - half-proudly.

There were several old cupboards in there with numerous boxes and one of them contained many faded wrinkled cartoons. I couldn't imagine that anybody could use those old things so I took his advice and threw everything out. Johnny came around a few days later and asked how everything was going. I told him I had cleared it all away, including the old cartoons which "you wouldn't want anyhow". He was polite and didn't say anything. Perhaps he had forgotten that the cartoons had ever been there.

Whenever we decided to work on something together he would say. "First we must talk about the title". So we sat there for 15 minutes and discussed it. Sometimes I would say, "I haven't any material. Do you really think it's worthwhile talking about it now"? "Definitely". Then every week over a cup of tea we would talk about the title. What it might be. What it could be. Who might be interested in reading the article or chapter or book. Looking back, I think he must have found this to be a way of relaxing and forgetting his fatigue and chronic pain.

When Johnny Lind embarked on his research on the fetal circulation, the human fetus was regarded as a placid, dependent, fragile vegetable who was developing in preparation for a life that would start after birth. Indeed, in the mid-1960s Johnny was still writing articles describing the fetus as a parasite and others were still using this term, even in 1978. Today the fetus, far from being regarded as an inert passenger in a pregnant mother, is seen as in command of the pregnancy. He does not live in a state of sensory deprivation but in a plastic, reactive structure which buffers and filters, and perhaps distorts, but does not eliminate the outside world. It would rather seem that it is the fetus who guarantees the endocrine success of pregnancy, who induces a number of changes in maternal physiology to make her a suitable host, who solves the homograft problem, and who determines the duration of pregnancy. When our cords are cut we are not severed from our mothers but from our own organs - our placentae - which are appropriate to our old environment but unnecessary in our new one. We do not regard the fetal circulatory system, different as it is from the child's or adult's, as one big agglomeration of congenital defects, but as a system superbly adapted to the environment in which the fetus lives.

The diagram shown here can be used to summarize some of Johnny's interests in the field of the fetal and neonatal circulation, ranging from studies on the placenta to the time of clamping of the umbilical cord, changes in the structure and function of the portal vein and the ductus venosus, the course of the circulation through the heart, some characteristics of the vessels leading to the brain, the initiation of the first breath, various aspects of adaptation of the kidney, anatomical differences between the inguinal vessels in infants with one or both of the umbilical arteries and the structure and closure mechanisms of the umbilical vessels (Fig 2).

One of the areas in which I worked while in Johnny Lind's department was pediatric electrocardiography. The change in attitude concerning the electrocardiogram of infants and children since the 1950s, at least in some respects, has been less dramatic than that about the fetus. One of the first books to be devoted solely to the subject

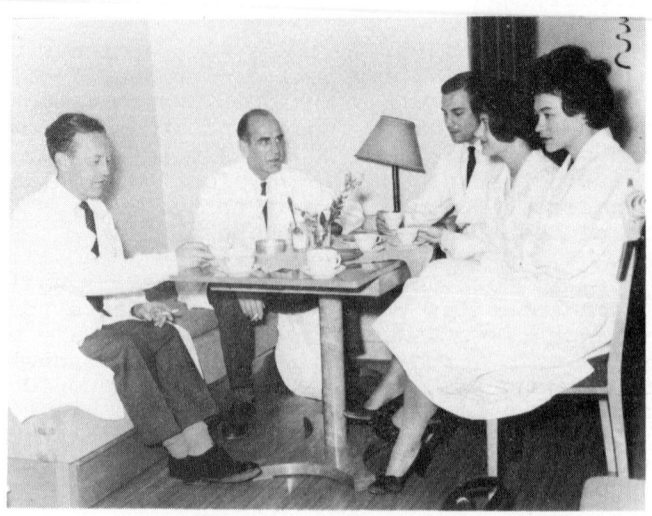

Fig. 1 Professor John Lind is seated at the end of the sofa on the far left side of the photograph. On his right is Dr. John R. Roberts of Liverpool, and on his left Dr. F. Michael Shepard of Johnson City, Tenn., Child Nurse, Mrs. Siv Lundqvist and Dr. Z. Walsh. Taken at a Stockholm Maternity Hospital (Södra B.B.) in mid-1960s.

of pediatric electrocardiography was written by Gertrude Nicolson in 1953. She stated in the introduction that "the normal electrocardiogram of a child", and I quote, "can be recognized by the <u>absence</u> of abnormal signs rather than by the <u>presence</u> of any definite characteristics". In 1965 Ziegler tried to reconcile reported differences in the electrocardiographic findings in infants by suggesting that it would be better to analyze the various studies and to determine what the differences in method were and why the findings were being interpreted differently.

There can be little question about the inportance of technically satisfactory fast multi-channel recordings, careful standardization and the accurate placement of electrodes. But there is some question whether it is possible to accurately select by palpation chest electrode positions in the infant. By convention, the angle of Louis (or Ludwig) is used as a convenient bony reference for counting the intercostal spaces. It is formed by the junction of the manubrium with the body of the sternum and located immediately above the second intercostal space. In one study tiny metal markers were placed on the chest at the site of lead V4 in one group of infants and on the nipple in another group of infants. Roentgenograms of the chest in frontal view were taken with both arms at the sides in order to avoid shifting of the nipple and they were interpreted by a well-known roentgenologist. It was found that the electrode on the nipple was more frequently located over the fifth intercostal space than was the electrode position selected by palpation. In fact, in the majority of cases the technician, who was very experienced, was unable, by palpation, to place the electrode over the fifth intercostal space. This is because it may be difficult, or even impossible, to palpate the angle of Louis in infants,

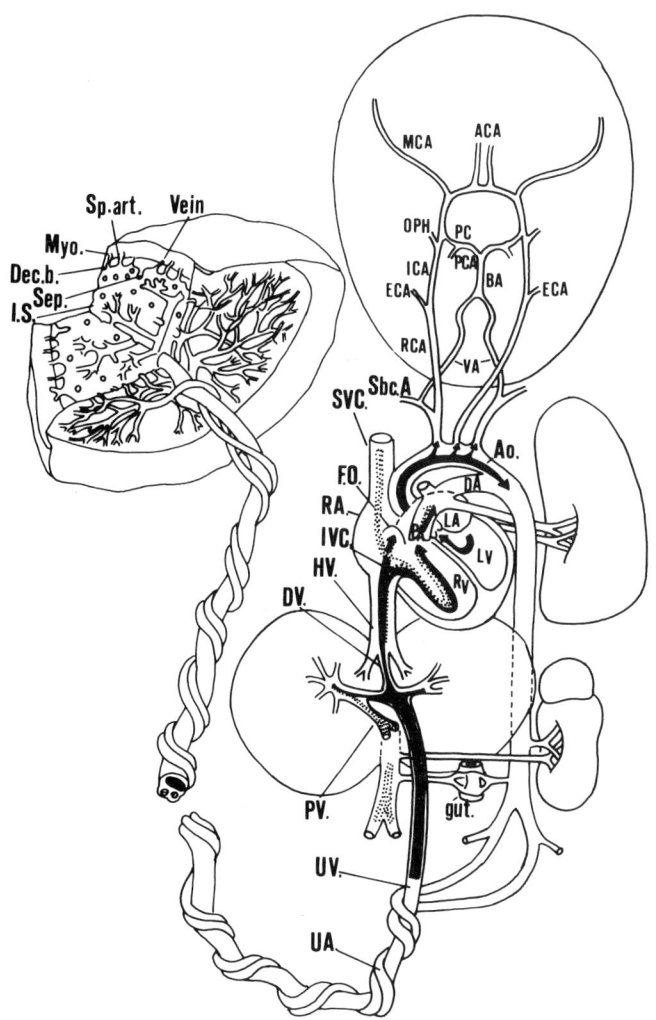

Fig. 2. Diagram showing the course of the fetal circulation.
(From Walsh, Meyer and Lind, 1974).

It is particularly important to determine the position of lead V4 correctly, since this is used to determine other electrode positions. The same applies to the recording of vectorcardiograms with the Frank system, in which all the five chest positions are located at the level of the fifth intercostal space. Therefore it seems reasonable that when the angle of Louis is hard to feel, the nipple should be the point of reference for selection of the electrode positions, at least in infants. Moreover, the nipple only rarely - i.e., in conditions such as bilateral renal hypoplasia and gonadal dysgenesis - has been reported to show a significant lateral displacement in relation to the mid-clavicular line.

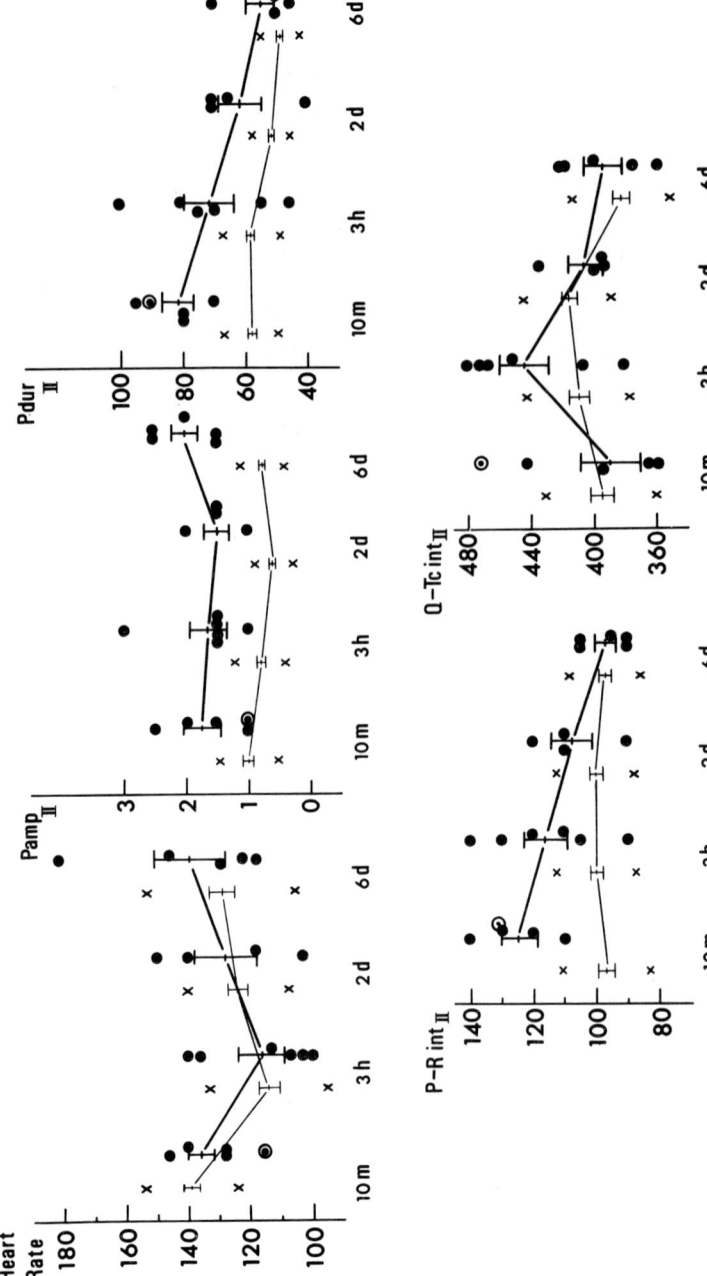

Fig. 3. Serial ECG findings in 31 infants with early clamping (light lines) and in 6 infants with vigorous stripping of the cord (heavy lines) during the first week of life. Note the higher P amplitude (Pamp), longer P-R and Q-Tc intervals, particularly on the first day in infants with stripping. ●: individual values in infants with stripping. ⊙: 45-minute old infant not included in mean. Mean (—), SE (=), and SD (X) are shown. (From Walsh, 1969).

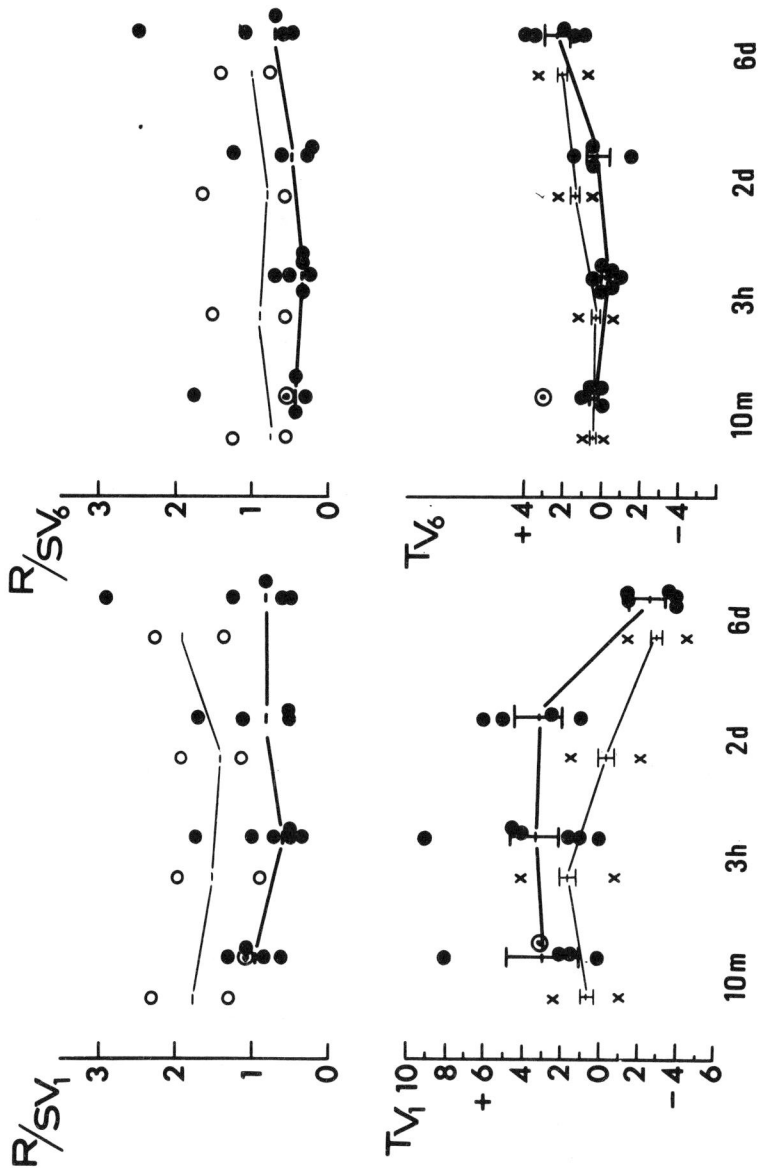

Fig.4. R/S and T in leads V1 and V6 in 31 infants with immediate clamping of the cord (light lines) and in 6 infants with stripping of the cord (heavy lines) during the first week. The median (———) and quartiles (○) are shown in early clamped infants and median (———) and individual values (●) in stripped cord infants for the R/S; the mean, SE and SD are shown for the T wave. Note LOWER R/S ratios and delayed inversion of T_{V1} in infants with stripping (From Walsh, 1969).

Fig. 5. Lead II recorded at 50 minutes after birth.
The heart rate has increased only very slightly but the P wave duration and P-R interval have both decreased with age.

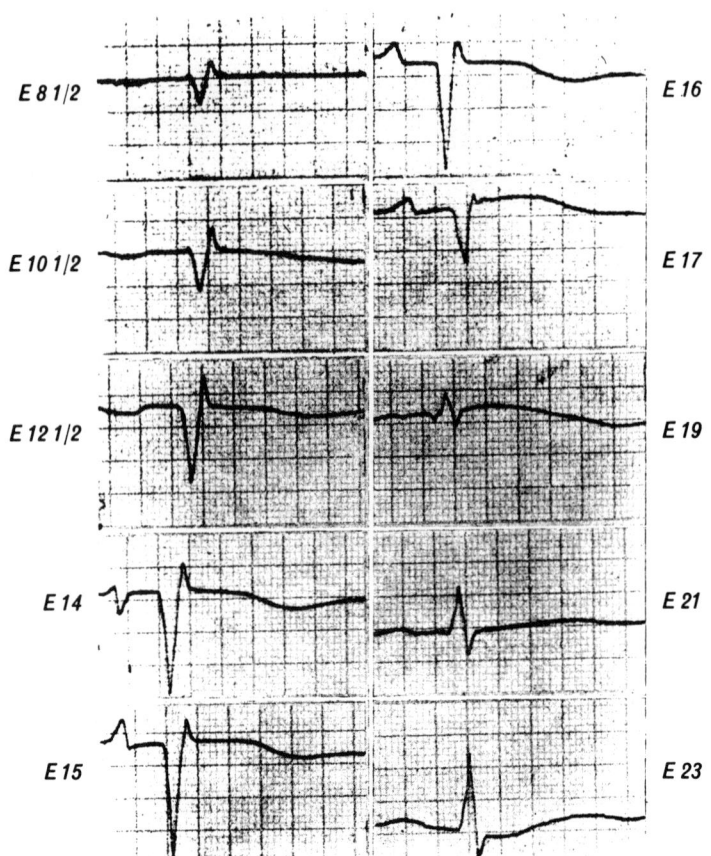

Fig. 6. Esophageal leads in a healthy 50-minute-old infant. Note P wave at E 14-15 is of relatively low amplitude at this age and shows sharp intrinsic deflection. In comparison to lead II, however, the P wave is well seen (see Fig.5 .) These two leads are designated as atrial, while those recorded above and below this area are referred to as supra- and infra-atrial respectively. The QRS complex in high leads generally resembles aVR while that in low leads resembles II or aVF (Recorded at 100 mm./sec.). Distance between fine horizontal lines = 1 mm.

In infancy, numerous changes in complexes are seen. These are undoubtedly due in part to complex alterations in the relation between electrode positions and the heart. Thus during the first year of life, the external dimensions of the thorax show a 30 to 50 per cent increase, and a change occurs in the relation of chest breadth to chest depth. Hence, prior to birth the chest on cross-section at the level of the nipples has the form of a slightly flattened oval and the depth of the chest equals about 85 per cent of its breadth. About 15 minutes after birth this value changes to 106 per cent because the A-P distance becomes much greater than the side- to-side distance. Not until the infant is about 2 1/2 months old does the value return to the prenatal level. At one year it is about 78 per cent. During the same period there is a marked retardation in the lateral extension of the nipple. The flattening of the chest wall and the changes in its dimensions also probably show considerable individual variations. Such variations undoubtedly affect the location of chest electrode positions in an unpredictable fashion.

Some insight into the electrocardiogram of the "healthy" fetus and neonate has been derived from various studies:

In the fetus:
1. Injection of oxygenated heparinized blood temporarily reverses the prolongation of electrocardiographic intervals which occurs immediately after delivery (Westin and Enhörning, 1955).
2. Clamping of the cord in utero causes an immediate and striking increase in amplitude of the Q and R waves in lead V1 among other changes (Stern et al., 1961).
3. But there is no relation between the height of the R wave and the thickness of the heart wall (at least in studies of epicardial excitation of the revived human fetal heart). Thus right ventricular hypertrophy cannot account for these experimental findings but a sudden reduction in oxygen supply, among other factors, can. In the term infant shortly after delivery:
1. Withdrawal of 10% of the estimated blood volume shortens the intervals (P, P-R, QRS, Q-Tc) and lowers the deflections (P, Q, R, S and T).
2. Reinjection of the same amount of blood largely reverses these effects. However, the effect on the Q-Tc cannot always be predicted.
3. Similar findings are obtained by clamping the cord early or vigorously milking it towards the infant. It is interesting in this connection that P amplitude differences are marked and are highly significant throughout the first week of life (Figs 3, 4)
4. A direct correlation exists between heart volume, determined on roentgenograms of the chest, and R and S waves in the right and left precordial leads but there is no such correlation with P amplitude, even in esophageal leads where they are best seen, or with various intervals (P, QRS or Q-Tc). (Figs 5, 6)
5. Higher pulmonary arterial pressures after birth show a direct correlation with higher P waves and upright T waves in lead V1.
6. Systolic blood pressures show a direct correlation with T waves in lead V5 at the end of the first week but no correlation with P amplitude or P duration.
7. Atrial pressures show no correlation with P wave amplitudes, even in esophageal leads.
8. The administration of glucose transiently affects the direction of T waves in precordial leads.

9. Body temperature shows an inverse correlation with the duration of the Q-Tc interval.
10. In infants who show an unusually high or low ratio of the P duration to the P-R segment, which Macruz interprets as a sign of left or right atrial enlargement, respectively - the ratio has a direct correlation with heart volume and systolic blood pressure as well as with the amplitude of various deflections in the left and right precordial leads.

Thus changes in blood volume are important in the genesis of changes in the electrocardiogram of the neonate. They also affect pressures and heart volume. However a host of other factors are undoubtedly involved. I believe that some of the above-mentioned studies help to explain the normal pattern of change in the electrocardiogram after birth which has been described by various authors. This pattern includes initially prolonged intervals (P, P-R, QRS, Q-Tc), initially increased R and S deflections over the right and mid-precordium, the gradual inversion of T waves over the right precordium, and the increasing amplitude of the Q, R, S and T waves over the left precordium towards the end of the first week.

REFERENCES

1. Nicolson G. H. B. (1953): Clinical Electrocardiography in Children, New York: MacMillan Co.
2. Stern, L. Lind, J., and Kaplan,B. (1961): Direct human fetal electrocariogaphy with studies of the effects of adrenalin, atropine, clamping of the umbilical cord and placental separation on the fetal ECG. Biol. Neonate 3,49.
3. Walsh, S. Z. (1969): Early clamping versus stripping of the cord. A comparative study of the electrocardiogram in the neonatal period. Brit.Heart J. 32, 122.
4. Walsh, S. Z., Meyer, W.W., and Lind, J. (1974): The Human Fetal and Neonatal Circulation: Function and Structure, Springfield, Ill.: Chas. C. Thomas.
5. Westin, B., and Enhörning, G. (1955): An experimental study of the human fetus with special reference to asphyxia neonatorum. Acta Paediat. Scand. 44,79.
6. Ziegler, R. F. (1965): Cardiac Evaluation in Normal Infants. Saint Louis, Mo.: C. V. Mosby Co.

RESUME.

Après une longue évocation de souvenirs personnels concernant Pr.John Lind, et un rappel de sa contribution fondamentale à la compréhension de la circulation foetale et de l'adaptation cardio-vasculaire à la vie extra-utérine, l'auteur décrit l'évolution de l'électrocardiographie pédiatrique depuis 1950 et ses propres recherches sur l'ECG du nouveau-né. En particulier, chez le nouveau-né à terme, peu après la naissance: 1) Un retrait de 10% du volume sanguin entraîne un raccourcissement des intervalles (P,P-R,QRS,Q-Tc) et une diminution des amplitudes (P,Q,R,S,T), effets abolis par la réinjection du même volume; 2) Des différences du même type sont observées entre les nouveau-nés ayant subi un clampage précoce du cordon ombilical et ceux ayant eu un clampage tardif avec essorage du cordon; 3) Il existe une corrélation directe entre le volume cardiaque (radiographie thoracique) et les amplitudes de R et S en dérivations précordiales; 4) La persistance de pressions pulmonaires élevées

s'accompagne d'ondes P plus amples et d'une onde T positive en V1;
5) La durée de l'intervalle Q-Tc est inversement proportionnelle à la température centrale.

Enfin, les variations de volume sanguin ont des répercussions notables sur l'ECG du nouveau-né, ainsi que sur les pressions et le volume cardiaque.

ST waveform analysis of the fetal ECG—a potent method for fetal surveillance? A presentation of experimental and clinical data

K.G. Rosén*, K.R. Greene§, K.-H. Hökegård†, K. Karlsson†, H. Lilja†, K. Lindecrantz‡ and I. Kjellmer*

Department of Pediatrics I*, Department of Physiology* and Department of Obstetrics and Gynecology†, University of Göteborg, Department of Applied Electronics‡, Chalmers University of Technology, Göteborg, Sweden and Nuffield Institute for Medical Research§, University of Oxford, England

ABSTRACT

Although considerable progress occurred with the introduction of electronic fetal monitoring it is now clear that fetal heart rate alone does not provide optimal information about the fetus. For the past ten years work by our group has been focused on the evaluation of ST waveform changes in the fetal ECG as a means for fetal surveillance. Fetal hypoxemia results in a reproducible pattern of changes with a progressive increase in T wave amplitude as the main response. The ratio between the amplitude of T wave and QRS complexe the T/QRS ratio, quantifies these T wave alterations.

Experiments on the acute fetal lamb and guinea-pig preparations have demonstrated a relationship between the breakdown of myocardial glycogen and high T waves, the development of a metabolic acidosis with increasing blood lactate and increased T/QRS ratios. The increase in T wave amplitude could be elicited by isoprenaline infusions and blocked by propranolol thus indicating that a beta-adrenergic mechanism is involved.

Furthermore the ST waveform changes appeared well in advance of any signs of cardio-vascular or cerebral collapse.

These studies have been carried on in the chronically catheterized fetal lamb preparation with the FECG recorded from a precordial lead. The data show an identical pattern of FECG change during maternally induced hypoxia with positive correlations between T/QRS and lactate ($r=0.784$, $p<0.001$) and between T/QRS and adrenaline ($r=0.765$, $p<0.001$).

During spontaneous labour in the chronic sheep ST waveform changes could appear for 12 hours before fetal death.

During human labour we are able to identify the same ST waveform changes from the scalp lead and a microprocessor based system has been developed for on line recording and quantification.

Keywords

Fetal asphyxia, fetal monitoring, fetal ECG, fetal sheep, human labour.

INTRODUCTION

Analysis of the waveform of the electrocardiogram (ECG) recorded during the perinatal period has been the subject of numerous studies over the part thirty years including those of John Lind and his associates (Stern and Lind, 1960; Stern, Lind and Kaplan, 1961). Most studies have used the human fetus investigating the possibility of early and safe diagnosis of fetal asphyxia. The introduction of electronic fetal monitoring was a considerable step forward in fetal surveillance but it is now clear that the fetal heart rate alone does not provide optimal information about the fetus. Thus, a question arises whether additional information could be gained by further analyzing the fetal ECG as this is likely to be the parameter presently most easily accessible during labour.

Over the past ten years our group has focused on the evaluation of ST waveform changes in the fetal ECG as a means of fetal surveillance. The ST interval represents repolarization of the myocardium which is an active metabolic process and more likely to be affected by alterations in cellular energy balance in the heart than e.g. the QRS complex.

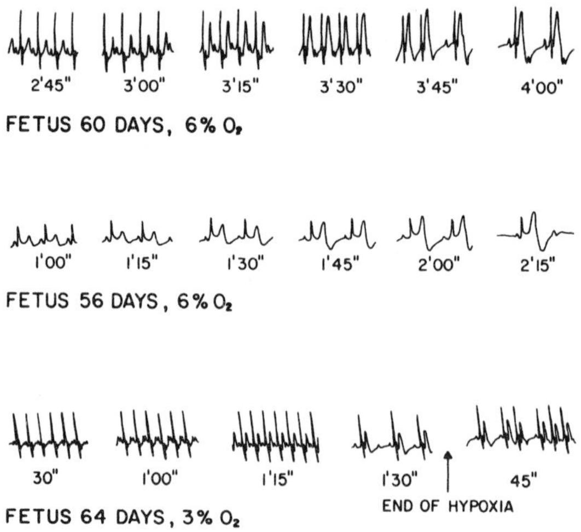

Fig. 1. Recordings of FECG from three guinea pig fetuses during hypoxia induced by ventilating the mother with 3 to 6 per cent O_2 (data from Rosén and Kjellmer, 1975).

The initial findings appeared during the study of the vagal influence on the fetal hypoxic bradycardia (Rosén and Kjellmer, 1975). These experiments were performed on the acutely exteriorized fetal guinea-pig preparation with crocodile clips applied over the precordium and on both forelegs to give a precordial ECG lead from which the fetal heart rate was calculated. Fig. 1 gives an example of FECG recordings during maternally induced hypoxia and ST waveform changes were identified in all cases in advance of any bradycardia.

Subsequent studies have been designed to evaluate the mechanisms of ST waveform change.

Studies have been done on both the acutely exteriorized as well as the chronically cannulated fetal sheep preparation. The former preparation will inevitably lead to fetal asphyxia but with good care there are at least three hours of a stable situation as judged by blood gases, cardiac output and plasma catecholamine levels (Rosén et al., to be published) and as our initial aim was to study fetal reactions to short-lasting asphyxic events we found the acutely exteriorized preparation suitable.

Sequence and quantification of ST waveform changes

Fig. 2 gives the whole sequence of ST waveform changes recorded from a mature fetal lamb. Alterations in the FECG were quantified according to a scoring system (Rosén and Isaksson, 1976) with the following definitions: **Grade I:** the appearance of negative T wave changes, the amplitude exceeding that of the P waves. **Grade II:** Maximally negative T wave changes. **Grade III:** A gradual decrease in the amplitude of the negative T wave changes. **Grade IV:** An elevation of the ST segment and the T wave, the amplitude of the T wave being higher than that of the P wave. **Grade V:** A maximal increase in the amplitude of the T wave. **Grade VI:** A decrease in the amplitude of the T wave during continuous hypoxia. This latter grade is a short-lasting event associated with bradycardia and cardiovascular collapse.

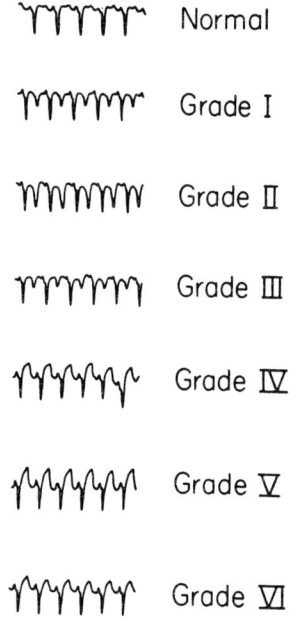

Fig. 2. The fetal ECG scoring system.

Since the predominant pattern seen is the progressive increase in T wave amplitude, the ratio between the amplitude of the QRS complex and the T wave (T/QRS ratio) was mainly used as quantitative measurement. The ratio was used rather than the absolute value of the T wave amplitude in order to eliminate the effects of difference in amplifications and as no alteration in QRS amplitude occurs (see Fig. 1, 2 and 5) a change in the ratio reflects an alteration in T wave amplitude. The T/QRS ratio could also be calculated by a computer and would serve as a more exact measurement than a scoring system.

ACUTELY EXTERIORIZED FETAL SHEEP

Metabolic relationships

The standard procedure to elicit hypoxia was to ventilate the ewe with a low oxygen containing gas mixture and take blood samples at 10 minutes intervals. Fig. 3 gives the relationship between pH and T/QRS ratio ($r=-0.86$, $p<0.001$). The graph also illustrates a upper level of normality in T/QRS ratio of around 0.3.

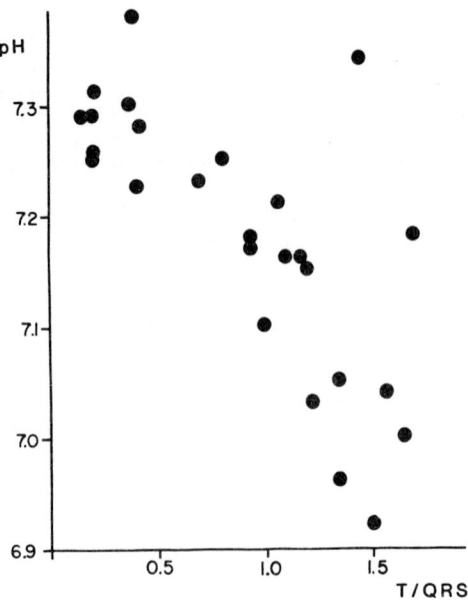

Fig. 3. The relationship between arterial pH and T/QRS ratio (data from Rosén et al., 1976).

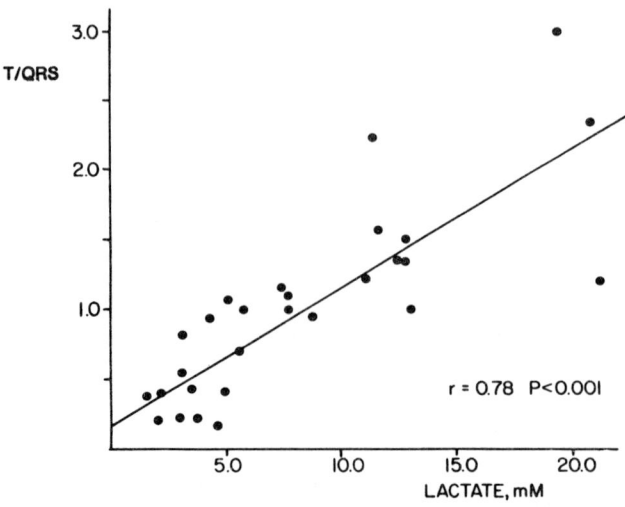

Fig. 4. Correlation between T/QRS ratio and blood lactate concentrations. The regression line is included (data from Rosén et al., 1976).

The acidosis was to a large extent due to an increase in blood lactate and an equally strong linear correlations was found between T/QRS and lactate concentrations (Fig. 4) (Rosén et al., 1976). This finding is of significance as it indicates a basic mechanism behind the ST waveform changes, namely the anaerobic breakdown of myocardial glycogen generating a surge of blood lactate (Dawes, Mott and Shelley, 1959). The myocardial metabolism has been directly studied during hypoxia and related to ST waveform changes. In the first study performed on mature guinea pig fetuses (Rosén and Isaksson, 1976) a linear relationship occurred between glycogen content of the fetal myocardium and the ST waveform changes during hypoxia. Myocardial ATP and creatine-phosphate were maintained until there were signs of myocardial failure with bradycardia (AV-block, type II). In this study each fetus gave one point of measurement during hypoxia and from each litter one fetus served as control and comparisons could be made during normoxia and hypoxia.

In the second study (Hökegård et al., 1981) repeated biopsies were taken from the epicardial surface of the working fetal heart at varying degrees of ST waveform changes during hypoxia. Wet weight concentrations of the organic muscle metabolites glycogen, CrP, ATP and lactate were determined with enzymatic assays. A linear decrease occurred in all energy rich substances during hypoxia. Glycogen content was reduced from 83.6 ± 9.6 mmol glucose/kg wet weight ($\pm$ SEM) to 30.0 ± 3.0 mmol glucose/kg w.w. when signs of failing cardiovascular functions appeared associated with Grade VI. This relationship between the utilization of myocardial glycogen and T wave amplitude was further strengthened when the rate of glycogenolysis was compared with the corresponding increase in T wave amplitude ($r=0.73$; $p<0.001$). Unless there were a marked acidosis, pH<7.04 and/or hypoglycemia the fetal myocardium was able to regenerate measurable amounts of glyocogen within 15 minutes.

Thus during a period of asphyxia a parallellity exists between myocardial glycogenolysis and increase in T wave amplitude. The importance of myocardial glycogenolysis as a major compensatory mechanism for the fetus during asphyxia is well known (Dawes, Mott and Shelley, 1959; Shelley, 1969) and any indicator of this would provide useful information about the fetal response to asphyxia.

The mechanism behind the ST waveform changes was further elucidated when the beta-adrenoceptor stimulating drug, isoprenaline, was given to the fetus and a dose response relationship was established (Hökegård et al., 1979). Adrenaline had previously been shown in human fetuses to elicite high T waves (Stern, Lind and Kaplan, 1961) and beta-adrenoceptor activation is known to induce glycogenolysis (Mayer et al., 1967). Thus, it appeared likely that the known adrenaline surge during hypoxia (Comline, Silver and Silver, 1965; Jones and Robinson, 1975) could be a factor responsible for the fetal ST waveform changes. The beta-adrenoceptor blocking drug, propranolol, was also shown to inhibit the ST changes during moderate hypoxia but ($P_{O_2}>1.5$ KPa) these changes remained during marked hypoxia. This is in keeping with the hypothesis that these FECG changes reflect myocardial glycogenolysis as hypoxia _per se_ is known to induce glycogenolysis (Mayer et al., 1967).

Relationship to cerebral and cardiovascular functions

We have used the somato-sensory evoked EEG potentials (SEP) as a measure of functional cortical activity. Alterations in SEP and FECG were found to be contemporaneous during the progression of asphyxia (Rosén et al., 1976). Furthermore the ST waveform changes occurred well in advance of any signs of deteriorating cardiovascular functions (Rosén, Hökegård and Kjellmer, 1976). During the marked hypoxic events that occurred in the acutely exteriorized preparation a parallellity often exist between an increase in T wave amplitude, increase in myocardial contractility, measured from a intraventricular micro-tip sensitive catheter and a tachycardia, all signs of cardiac effects of an increase in sympathetic tone. As the ST waveform changes could be induced, not only during hypoxia but also during normoxia in the latter case in combination with signs of an increase in myocardial performance (increased contractility and tachycardia) the assumption was made that the T/QRS ratio could serve as an index of myocardial energy balance.

CRONICALLY CANNULATED FETAL SHEEP

In the process of evaluating any method for fetal surveillance maximal information should preferably be gained before starting a clinical trial.

The chronically instrumented fetal sheep preparation would be a most valuable complement as external influences on the preparation should be minimal and the initial work was started in 1977 at the Nuffield Institute for Medical Research, Oxford (Greene et al., 1983) and was carried on in Göteborg (Rosén et al., 1984).

The hypoxia was instituted by letting the ewe breath a 7-9% oxygen containing gas mixture for one hour.

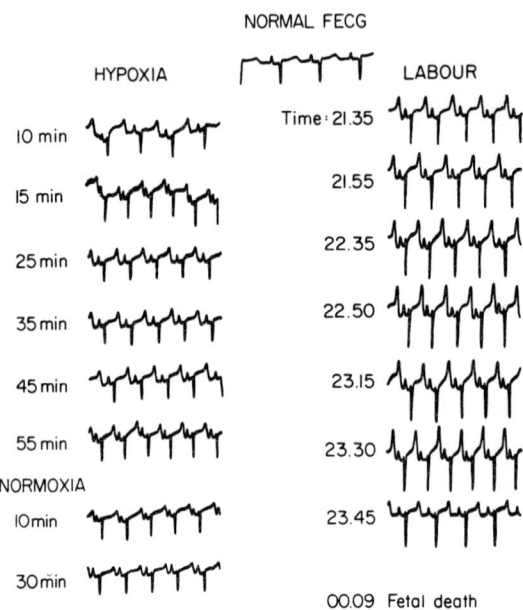

Fig. 5. Fetal ECG recordings from a chronically catheterized fetal sheep subjected to 60 minutes of hypoxia. The graph also indicates ST waveform changes appearent during labour and preceeding death by hours.

Figure 5 gives an example of ST waveform changes emerging during this hypoxic procedure. Evidently the same type of FECG changes, as previously studied during the exteriorized condition, could be recorded. However, there were periods when the ewe was allowed to breathe the hypoxic gas mixture where no ST waveform changes occurred. In this group of fetuses pH as well as lactate was normal, 7.35 ± 0.02 and 1.94 ± 0.54 mmol/l (mean $\pm$ SD) during the experiment. In the hypoxic experiments with substantial changes in the ST waveform (T/QRS exceeding 0.3 and increasing from 0.17 ± 0.05 to 0.59 ± 0.31; $\pm$ SD, $p<0.01$) all variables measured except P_{CO_2} and fetal heart rate showed a statistically significant change. the largest change was in blood lactate concentrations, from 1.15 ± 0.44 to 8.08 ± 3.86 mmol/l ($p<0.001$). There was also a rise in fetal glucose concentration, 1.04 ± 0.49 to 1.98 ± 0.53 mmol/l, a fall in pH from 7.36 ± 0.03 to 7.28 ± 0.10 and an increase in mean arterial pressure from 49.3 ± 7.9 to 58.9 ± 7.1 mm Hg. Judging from these data hypoxic periods with ST waveform changes ment a hypoxic insult to the fetus although adequately handled. During hypoxic periods without ST waveform changes the metabolic effect of the hypoxia was likely to be within the limits of normal aerobic cellular metabolism.

A multiple correlation analysis was performed on 37 sets of observation with T/QRS ratio as the dependent variable. The strongest correlation was found between T/QRS and blood lactate ($r=0.784$, $p<0.001$). This relationship was further strengthened when relating the T/QRS ratio to the rate of lactate rise during the preceeding 20 minutes ($r=0.815$). Thus, these data complemented and strengthened the data obtained from the acutely exteriorized and anesthetized fetal sheep.

Circulating catecholamines

A further piece of information was added when the surge of cathecolamines was measured and related to the ST waveform changes during one hour hypoxic period (Rosén et al., 1984). The findings were identical of those in the previous study with hypoxic periods showing no T wave changes as well as those with marked alterations. In the previous case oxygen content fell by 64% to 27.8 ± 14.1 ml oxygen/l (P_{O_2} 1.72 ± 0.20 kPa) yet no adrenaline was released. With the appearance of T wave changes a substantial release of adrenaline occurred from 1.84 (median, range 0-9.97 nmol/l) to 22.97, range 1.6-87.0 nmol/l. A linear correlation was also appearent between adrenaline concentrations and T/QRS ratio ($r=0.765$, $p<0.001$). Under these circumstances oxygen content had dropped to 19.8 ± 8.2 ml O_2/l (68%) and it is likely that the increase in myocardial blood flow induced by hypoxia would not compensate for the fall in oxygen content (Peeters et al., 1979) and anaerobic myocardial metabolism would occur with the appearance of high T waves.

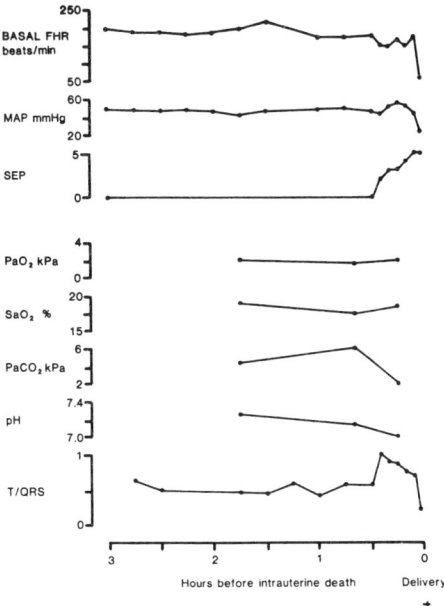

Fig. 6. Alterations in fetal heart rate, mean arterial blood pressure (MAP), somatosensory evoked EEG potentials (SEP), blood gases, oxygen saturation, pH and T/QRS ratio during the last three hours of labour at 143 days gestation, ending in fetal death at time of delivery. The SEP was recorded by a signal averager with EEG electrodes fixed over the suprasylvian gyrus on both sides and the somatosensory impuls evoked by mechanically stimulate the nostril area on one side. A scoring system was used for SEP quantification with Grade 0 as the normal response and Grade V as no response at all (data from Rosén et al., 1985).

LABOUR RECORDINGS - SHEEP

All studies performed so far included artificially induced hypoxia. The chronically cannulated fetal sheep preparations allows recordings to be undertaken during spontaneous labour and delivery. Our initial observations has been reported (Rosén et al., 1985) and includes two fetuses entering labour at 125 and 143 days gestation. In these two cases we were able to include somatosensory evoked EEG responses (SEP) from the fetus from start of labour to time of fetal death. Fig. 6 shows the recordings made during the last three hours of labour in the mature fetus. The fetal brain showed a remarkable capacity to maintain its functional integrity and not until the last 30 minutes a rapid deterioration occurred with brain death 6 min before the last heart beat. Labour had been in progress for 32 hours and significant ST waveform changes occurred during the last 12 hours of labour with a progressive increase in T wave amplitude in parallel with an increase in uterine activity and the degree of hypoxia. Bradycardia and fall in blood pressure appeared during the last five minutes in parallel with a decrease in T/QRS ratio that would correspond to Grade VI of the scoring system. Thus, the return in T wave amplitude during continuous asphyxia is a late event associated with other signs of cardiovascular collaps. Furthermore, ST waveform changes preceed hypoxic alterations in fetal cerebral cortical acitivity as measured from somatosensory evoked EEG responses during intrauterine circumstances. Thus, experimental data have provided a parameter which could be of high clinical relevance and the state of knowledge could thus be summarized:

A: METABOLIC RELATIONSHIPS

T/QRS ratio related to

1. The rate of myocardial glycogenolysis.
2. Circulating levels of adrenaline (beta-adrenoceptor stimulation).
3. A metabolic acidosis.
5. Reduction in PaO_2.

B: METHOD FOR FETAL MONITORING

T/QRS ratio

- indicates asphyxia prior to alteration in evoked EEG responses, a measure of functional cerebral activity
- appears in a advance of signs of cardiovascular failure and gives an estimation of myocardial energy balance.

LABOUR RECORDINGS - HUMAN

Any waveform analysis requires a stable signal with a high signal to noise level. Since the initial work by Hon (1963) the scalp electrode has provided a possibility although some additional technique, like signal averaging is needed both for the purpose of reducing noice (Fig. 7) and handling the large amount of data. Even with an optimal QRS detector, using a pattern recognition system (Lindecrantz, 1983), averaging could affect the information looked for as examplified by a false increase in T/QRS ratio due to a false decrease in QRS amplitude. Fig. 7 also denotes the effect of noise on the possibility to use an automatic assessment of T wave amplitude by calculating the T/QRS ratio. Thus, optimal signal quality is most essential in ST waveform analysis and all signal filters should be avoided. The only way to achieve this for the moment is to have direct fetal ECG electrodes applied to the presenting part of the fetus.

Another crucial question is the possiblity of T wave monitoring from a peripheral scalp electrode. Experimental data (Hökegård and Rosén, 1980) from the fetal sheep had demonstrated a possibility to detect T wave changes from electrodes placed over the

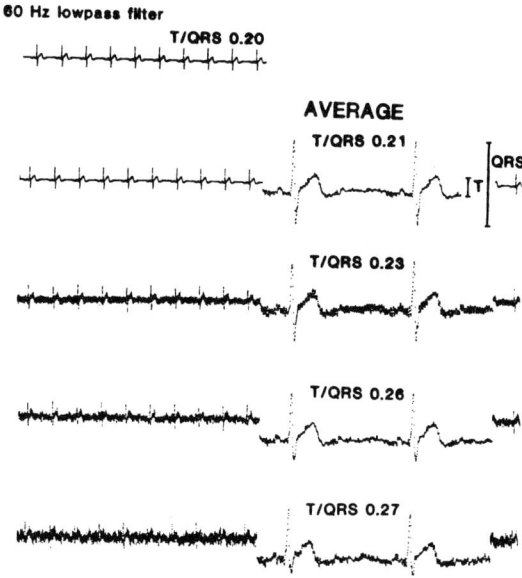

Fig. 7. The influence of signal filter, signal averaging and signal noise on the T/QRS ratio (data from Lindecrantz, 1983).

precordium and the scalp. This mode of FECG recording was mimiced clinically by recording a FECG during labour with the use of a catheter-tip electrode, placed down the back of the fetus (Fig. 8), and a scalp electrode (Lilja et al., 1985). The two exploring electrodes decreased baseline fluctuations as compared with the standard recording procedure with one scalp electrode.

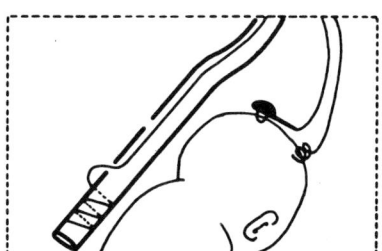

Fig. 8. An illustration of the fetal ECG electrodes and their relationship on the fetus.

Figure 9 illustrates the fetuses of one case with ST waveform changes through most of the labour. The mother, a primigravida with hypertension at term, was induced by intravaginal prostaglandin E_2 gel and developed uterine hypertonus with amniotic pressures of 20-25 mm Hg between contractions. The elevated T/QRS ratio varied between 0.57 and 1.12 with a noticeable increase with contractions and decrease between but also generally increasing as labour progressed. The CTG tracing showed mainly variable decelerations with periods of

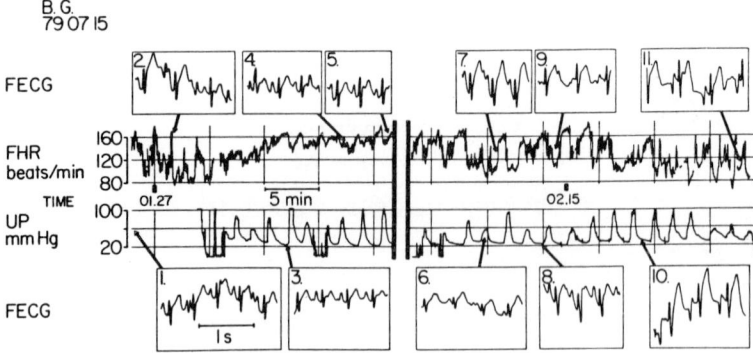

Fig. 9. Parallel recordings obtained of CTG and FECG during labour. Marked ST waveform changes visible throughout the recording. From 02.15 hrs the recording mode was altered from scalp-scalp to scalp-catheter electrodes (data from Lilja et al., 1985).

baseline bradycardia. The infant was delivered spontaneously with Apgar scores of 7 at one minute and 9 at five minutes. The umbilical artery pH was 7.24, the lactate 5.15 mmol/l and the neonatal period uneventful. From 02.15 hrs the recording method was changed from scalp-scalp to scalp-catheterelectrodes. Thus, it was obvious that ST waveform changes could be recorded by applying electrodes to the fetal scalp. This finding is further examplified in Fig. 10. This figure shows parallel ECG recordings from the fetal scalp lead and the precordial lead during the last stage of a sheep delivery. The FECG could be monitored from subcutaneously placed scalp electrodes due to the previous dissapearence of EEG activity. The impact of a 1 Hz high pass filter on ST waveform is also noticable.

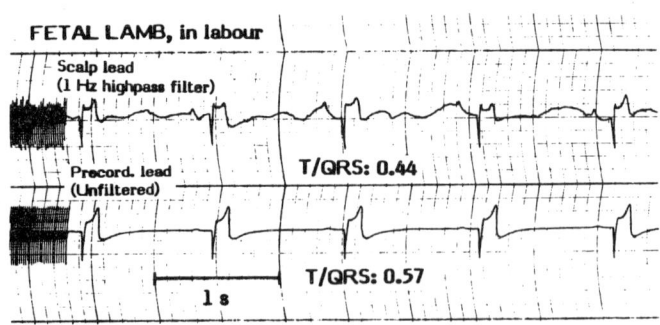

Fig. 10. Parallel recordings of FECG from scalp and precordial leads.

The question now to be asked is whether a breech delivery will give the same possiblity to detect any ST waveform changes. Figure 11 gives an exampel of ST waveform changes during breech delivery with an increase in T wave amplitude as the baby was born. So it appears possible to detect ST waveform changes not only from the fetal scalp but also from the fetal buttock.

76

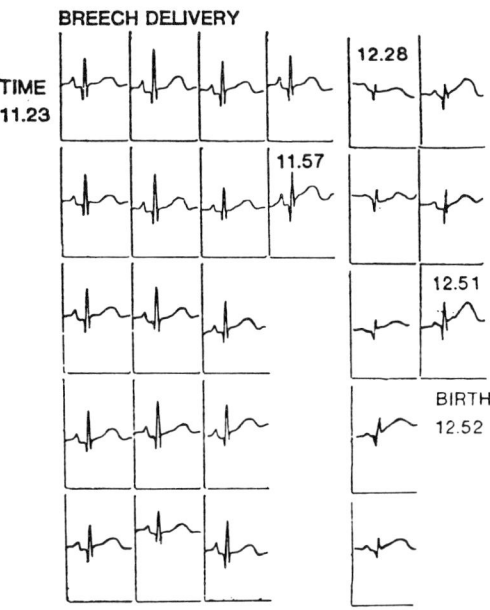

Fig. 11. The fetal ECG recorded during a breech delivery. Two vaginal electrodes were placed on the buttock and the signal was processed in an averaging system (Wickham, 1982). Note the increase in T wave amplitude prior to birth which was uneventful.

Table I. Relationship between T/QRS and classification of CTG.

Patients:	96 (1/3 at risk)
Outcome:	Apgar 5 min >7 in all cases
Emergency op. proc. due to fetal distress:	14 cases
Neonat. period:	VOC 1 case RDS 3 cases

T/QRS   C T G

	NORM	INTERMED	ABNORM	
<0.30	27	19	20	66
0.3–0.6	4	2	13	19
>0.60			2	2
ST-depr. neg T	1	6	1	8
	32	27	36	

Table II. Classification of intrapartum CTG

Class I Normal CTG

    Basal heart frequency 120-160 beats/minute
    Heart rate variability (band width) 10-25 beats/minute
    No decelerations*

Class II Intermediate CTG

    Basal heart frequency 100-120 or 160-180 beats/minute
    Heart rate variability (band width) >25 beats/minute
    Heart rate variability (band width) <5-10 beats/minute**
    Early decelerations in first stage
    Mild variable decelerations
        >80 beats/minute
        <60 seconds duration

Class III Abnormal CTG

    Basal heart frequency <100 or >180 beats/minute
    Heart rate variability (band width) <5 beats/minute in absence of sedation

    Moderate - severe variable decelerations
        <80 beats/minute
        >60 seconds duration

    Late decelerations

---

*)   early decelerations accepted as normal in second stage
**) band width 5-10 beats/minute accepted as normal together with accelerations.

T/QRS - CTG

We have so far discussed mainly methodological problems in assessing the ST waveform of the fetal ECG during labour. Our presently evaluated clinical data is summarized in Table I. The Table describes the relationship between CTG and max T/QRS ratio recorded during each delivery. With our previous knowledge from "chronic" fetal sheep a ratio of <0.3 is regarded as normal. A ratio between 0.3 and 0.6 would indicate a mild fetal hypoxia well compensated for and a ratio >0.6 could mean a more marked hypoxic insult. Only two babies had T/QRS ratios >0.6, one for a 20 minutes period (max T/QRS 0.85) and the other case is presented in Fig. 9.

This pattern of T/QRS ratios might well be in accordance with the complete lack of postnatal asphyxia among the babies.

The clinical situation during labour was that of abnormal CTG patterns (for definitions see Table II) in 38% of the patients and 15% had emergency operative deliveries due to "fetal distress". Lactate analysis were performed on cord blood from 41 cases showing all values <8 mmol/l.

From these data it is concluded that ST waveform analysis contains relevant information on the degree of fetal asphyxia that adds to the information obtained from the CTG recording. The final judgement could be made after a multicenter trial including clearly asphyxiated fetuses.

ACKNOWLEGEMENTS

These studies were supported by the Swedish Medical Research Council (grants no 5654 and 2591), the Medical Research Council of Great Britain, the "Expressen" Prenatal Research Foundation, Allmänna Barnbördshusets Memorial Foundation, the First of May Flower Annual Campaign for Childrens Health, the Medical Faculty, University of Göteborg and the Göteborg Medical Society.

REFERENCES

Comline, R.S., Silver, I.A. and Silver, M. (1965): Factors responsible for the stimulation of the adrenal medulla during asphyxia in the foetal lamb. **J. Physiol. 178:** 211.

Dawes, G.S., Mott, J.C. and Shelley, H.J. (1959): The importance of cardiac glycogen for the maintenance of life in foetal lambs and newborn animals during anoxia. **J. Physiol. 146:** 516.

Greene, K.R., Dawes, G.S., Lilja, H. and Rosen, K.G. (1982): Changes in the ST waveform of the fetal lamb electrocardiogram with hypoxia. **Amer. J. Obstet. Gynecol. 144:** 950.

Hon, E.H. (1963): Instrumentation of fetal heart rate and fetal electrocardiography. II. A vaginal electrode. **Am. J. Obstet. Gynecol. 86:** 772.

Hökegård, K.-H., Eriksson, B.O., Kjellmer, I., Magno, R. and Rosén, K.G. (1981): Myocardial metabolism in relation to electrocardiographic changes and cardiovascular function during graded hypoxia in the fetal lamb. **Acta Physiol. Scand. 113:** 1.

Hökegård, K.-H., Karlsson, K., Kjellmer, I. and Rosén, K.G.: ECG-changes in the fetal lamb during asphyxia in relation to beta-adrenoceptor stimulation and blockade. **Acta Physiol. Scand. 105:** 195.

Jones, C.T. and Robinson, R.O. (1975): Plasma catecholamines in foetal and adult sheep. **J. Physiol. 248:** 15.

Lilja, H., Greene, K.R., Karlsson, K. and Rosen, K.G. (1985): ST waveform changes of the fetal electrocardiogram during labour. A clinical study. **Br. J. Obstet. Gynaecol.** In press.

Lindecrantz, K. (1983): Processing of the fetal ECG: An implementation of a dedicated real time microprocessor system. **Technical Report No 135,** Chalmers University of Technology, Göteborg, Sweden.

Mayer, S.E., Williams, B.J. and Smith, J.M. (1967): Adrenergic mechanisms in cardiac glycogen metabolism. **Ann. N.Y. Acad. Sci. 139:** 686.

Peeters, L.L., Sheldon, R.E., Jones, M.D., Makowski, E.L. and Meschia, G. (1979): Blood flow to fetal organs as a function of arterial oxygen content. **Am. J. Obstet. Gynecol. 135:** 637.

Rosén, K.G., Dagbjartsson, A., Henriksson, B.-Å., Lagercrantz, H. and Kjellmer, I. (1984): The relationship between circulating catecholamines and ST waveform in the fetal lamb electrocardiogram during hypoxia. **Amer. J. Obstet. Gynecol. 149:** 190.

Rosén, K.G., Hrbek, A., Karlsson, K., Kjellmer, I., Olsson, T. and Riha, M. (1976): Changes in the ECG and somatosensory evoked EEg responses during intrauterine asphyxia in the sheep. **Biol. Neonate 30:** 95.

Rosén, K.G., Hökegård, K.-H. and Kjellmer, I. (1976): A study of the relationship between the electrocardiogram and hemodynamics in the fetal lamb during asphyxia. **Acta physiol. scand. 98:** 275.

Rosén, K.G. and Isaksson, O. (1976): Alterations in fetal heart rate and ECG correlated to glycogen, creatine phosphate and ATP levels during graded hypoxia. **Biol. Neonate 30:** 17.

Rosén, K.G., Lilja, H., Hökegård, K.-H. and Kjellmer, I. (1985): The relationship between cerebral cardiovascular and metabolic functions during labour in the lamb fetus. Symposium on the Physiological Development of the Fetus and Newborn. Academic Press, London (ed. C.T. Jones).

Rosén, K.G. and Kjellmer, I. (1975): Changes in the fetal heart rate and ECG during hypoxia. **Acta Physiol. Scand. 93:** 59.

Shelley, H.J. (1961): Glycogen reserves and their changes at birth and in anoxia. **Brit. Med. Bull. 17:** 137.

Stern, L. and Lind, J. (1960): The electrocardiogram at birth. **Biol. Neonate 2:** 34.

Stern, L., Lind, J. and Kaplan, B. (1961): Direct human foetal electrocardiography (with studies of the effect of adrenaline, atropine, clamping the umbilical cord, and placenta separation on the foetal ECG). **Biol. Neonate 3:** 49.

Wickham, P.J.D. (1982): Microprocessor based signal averager for analysis of the foetal ECG. **Med. Biol. Eng. and Comp. 3:** 253.

RESUME

L'introduction du monitorage électronique foetal a représenté un progrès considérable. Toutefois il s'avère maintenant que la seule fréquence cardiaque foetale n'apporte pas une information optimale sur l'état du foetus. Au cours de la dernière décennie, cette équipe s'est centrée sur l'évaluation des modifications de ST sur l'électrocardiogramme foetal (ECGF), comme moyen de surveillance du foetus. L'hypoxémie foetale s'accompagne d'un mode reproductible de variations de l'ECGF, dont la principale est une augmentation progressive de l'amplitude de l'onde T (voir figure 2). Ces altérations de l'onde T peuvent être quantifiées, en calculant le rapport de l'amplitude de T à l'amplitude du complexe QRS (qui ne change pas), à savoir le rapport T/QRS.

En expérimentation aiguë sur le foetus extériorisé d'agneau, l'hypoxie foetale est obtenue en ventilant la mère-brebis avec un mélange à faible FiO2. On met alors en évidence une corrélation entre le pH foetal et le rapport T/QRS, le développement d'une acidose métabolique avec augmentation des lactates sanguins foetaux et l'élévation du rapport T/QRS. Des microbiopsies myocardiques prélevées à différents stdes d'altération de ST ont montré une décroissance linéaire de tous les substrats énergétiques au cours de l'hypoxie, avec une corrélation entre le catabolisme du glycogène myocardique et l'élévation de T ($r = 0,73$; p inférieur à $0,001$). Cette augmentation d'amplitude de T peut aussi être obtenue par perfusion d'isoprénaline, et bloquée par administration de propanolol (du moins en hypoxie modérée, non en hypoxie majeure), ce qui indique la mise en jeu d'un mécanisme béta-adrénergique.

De plus, les modifications de ST apparaissent bien avant tout signe
de défaillance cardio-vasculaire ou d'altération cérébrale (mesure
de l'activité corticale par enregistrement des potentiels évoqués
somato-sensoriels).

Des travaux similaires ont été menés sur des foetus d'agneau
cathétérisés en préparation chronique, avec enregistrement de l'ECGF
à partir d'une électrode précordiale. Les données montrent un mode
identique de variation de l'ECGF au cours d'une hypoxie induite en
faisant respirer une FiO2 de 7-9% à la brebis pendant une heure. Il
existe des corrélations positives entre le rapport T/QRS et le taux
des lactates plasmatiques foetaux (r= 0,784; p inférieur à 0,001) et
entre T/QRS et le taux d'adrénaline circulante (r=0,765; p inférieur
à 0,001).

Sur une préparation chronique, lorsque la brebis entre en travail,
les modifications foetales de ST peuvent apparaître jusqu'à 12
heures avant la mort du foetus.

Au cours du travail chez la femme, les mêmes modifications de ST ont
été observées sur les ECGF obtenus à partir d'électrodes fixées sur
le cuir chevelu du foetus. En présentation du siège, la méthode
semble utilisable en fixant les électrodes sur le siège du foetus.
Un système incluant un microprocesseur permet la quantification en
temps réel et l'enregistrement. L'analyse de ST apporte alors des
éléments supplémentaires permettant de nuancer l'évaluation fournie
par les données cardio-tocographiques.

****

DISCUSSION. Dr.L.Stern, moderator.

Dr.J.Warshaw: Can you tell us how you sampled tissue?

Dr.K.Rosen: We opened the thorax and by a small hole we took tissue
samples of about 3 milligrams.

Dr.Ab.Rudolph: I would like to comment about changes in oxygenation
of the fetal myocardium. Studies we have done recently (Slate K,
Mills A, & Rudolph A. Unpublished observations) have shown that the
fetal myocardium has remarkable reserve in response to fetal
asphyxia. When we acutely reduced arterial oxygen saturation to
levels of 25 per cent, fetal myocardial oxygen consumption was
maintained because there was a huge increase in myocardial blood
flow. I suspect that the EKG changes described more likely result
from the effects of catecholamines. Some years ago, in studies in
adult dogs, I observed that infusion of epinephrine into a small
coronary artery resulted in changes in the surface electrogram
recorded from the heart in the region perfused (unpublished
observations)

Dr.K.Rosen: The following figure illustrates what I think are the
main events during hypoxia with a stimulation of the aortic chemoreceptor leading to catecholamine surge, which is a main fetal
compensatory response. An adrenaline surge is likely to increase the
myocardial performance and thereby to alter the energy balance over
the myocardium, resulting in myocardial glycogenolysis and ST
waveform changes. The adrenaline effect seems to operate over the
beta-adrenoreceptors, as ST waveform changes could be blocked by the
non-selective blocking drug, propanolol. This blocking effect was not

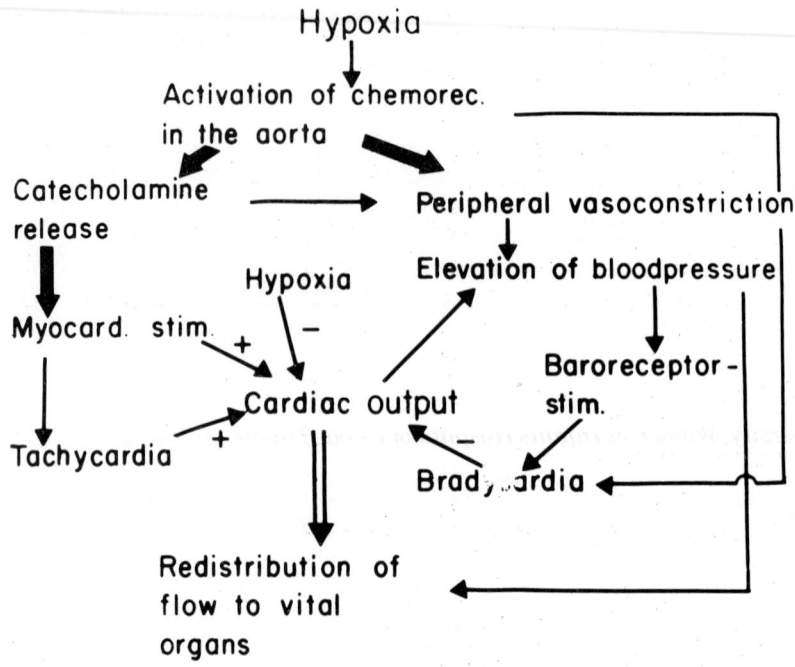

absolute as severe hypoxia per se could induce the EKG changes, probably by direct stimulation of glycogenolytic activity.

Dr. Ab. Rudolph: I believe that the changes you describe are probably rather the result of a membrane effect of catecholamines, because the ST and T wave changes are similar to those we saw with intra-coronary infusion of epinephrine. I do not believe they are caused by metabolic effects of hypoxia.

Dr. J. Warshaw: Have you looked at creatine phosphate or ATP levels as an index of energy reserve in the heart?

Dr. K. Rosen: Among the energy-rich purines, ATP stores were depleted in an almost linear fashion with the progress of hypoxia and the increasing FEKG scores. Creatine-phosphate on the other hand followed a more unpredictable pattern with a 50 per cent depletion during the initial phase of hypoxia. This level was then maintained.

Neonatal polycythaemia and hyperviscosity: the pathophysiological role of placental transfusion

W. Oh

Brown University, Women & Infants Hospital of Rhode Island, 50 Maude Street, Providence, Rhode Island 02908, USA

ABSTRACT

Polycythemia and hyperviscosity in the newborn are common disorders and the complexity and non specificity of the symptom complex is probably related to the multifactorial events that lead to the development of neonatal polycythemia and hyperviscosity. The role of placental transfusion both *in utero* and during the immediate postnatal period can account for many of these phenomenae on the basis of physiologic adaptation in response to acute expansion of blood volume.

KEY WORDS

Polycythemia, hyperviscosity, placental transfusion, blood volume, neonatal adaptation, delayed cord clamping.

INTRODUCTION

Polycythemia and hyperviscosity is a common problem in the newborn period. The incidence is variable ranging as high as 5% in the study conducted in Denver, Colorado, and 2.7% in Virginia (Wirth et al. 1979; Stevens & Wirth, 1980). The high incidence in the Colorado Study has been attributed to the fact that infants born at high altitudes will have an increase in fetal erythropoiesis. It is also recognized that other factors may influence the incidence of polycythemia and hyperviscosity, most strikingly, the effect of placental transfusion as evidenced from some earlier reports on the occurrence of plethora or polycythemia resulting from maternal fetal transfusion (Minkowski, 1962) or fetal to fetal transfusions (Widness et al., 1981). It is apparent that since blood volume *in utero* is in one compartment with two-thirds of the fetal placental blood volume being in the fetus and the remaining third in the placenta, any blood volume redistribution under a variety of circumstances can influence the ultimate blood volume both *in utero* and immediately after birth. If the redistribution results in transfer of blood from the placental to the fetal circuits, and if the transfer takes place acutely, a sudden expansion of the fetal blood volume will necessitate a physiologic readjustment until the circulating blood volume is balanced with the fetal or neonatal circulatory capacity. The physiologic adaptation occurs most dramatically after birth following the placental transfusion by delayed cord clamping in the vaginally delivered infant with a gravity gradient favoring the continuing flow of blood through the umbilical vein into the fetus. The adjustment occurs primarily through transcapillary movement of fluid into the extravascular space resulting in a reduction of blood volume, plasma volume and a concomitant rise of hematocrit. The rise in hematocrit may exceed normal range resulting in polycythemia and hyperviscosity. The purpose of this report is to present evidence to support this contention and elaborate on the role of placental transfusion in the clinical-pathophysiologic correlation of infants with polycythemia and hyperviscosity.

PATHOPHYSIOLOGIC CONSEQUENCE OF FETAL BLOOD VOLUME CHANGES

Figure 1 shows the proposed pathophysiologic role of changes in fetal blood volume and neonatal polycythemia and hyperviscosity. During pregnancy, several high risk events such as poorly controlled diabetes, preeclampsia, chronic hypertension, etc. may produce chronic fetal hypoxemia. There is good evidence that show infants born to these high risk mothers have elevated cord blood erythropoietin (Widness et al., 1&91; Finne, 1966). Erythropoietin is a hormone responsible for the induction of erythropoiesis. It is, therefore, very likely that when fetal hypoxia occurs with an elevation of erythropoietin, increase in placental-fetal blood volume may take place as a result of increase in erythropoiesis. If complications arise during labor resulting in fetal hypoxia, there will be a redistribution of blood volume resulting in a transfer of blood from the placental to the fetal compartment. In other words, acute hypoxia in utero in the presence of intact umbilical circulation may result in intrauterine placental transfusion with a reduction in placental blood volume and an increase in fetal blood volume. Evidence for this phenomenon is available both in the animal model as well as in human studies. In a study conducted by Oh et al.(1975), blood volume in the placenta and fetus were determined in chronically instrumented fetal lambs. When 30 minutes of fetal hypoxia was induced by maternal hypoxia, a 27 per cent increase in fetal blood volume (86 ± 3 to 108 ± 7 ml/kg body weight) was observed with a reciprocal reduction in placental blood volume (Figure 2). In human infants, three studies (Philip et al. 1969; Flod & Ackerman, 1971; Yao & Lind, 1972) have shown that perinatal asphyxia results in intrauterine placental transfusion resulting in an increase in fetal blood volume. Figure 3 shows the data of Yao and Lind which indicate a similar percentage in the increase in fetal blood volume (25%) in infants with perinatal asphyxia as those seen in chronic lamb studies (Oh et al.,1975).

The phenomenon of postnatal placental transfusion as a function of delayed clamping of the umbilical cord is well known. When an infant is born vaginally and placed approximately 10 to 15 cm below the birth canal, a sustained umbilical venous blood flow with a reduction in umbilical arterial blood flow returning to the placenta will result in a net increase in neonatal blood volume. Several studies have been performed to confirm this phenomenon and it is nicely summarized by Yao and Lind (1982).

While chronic increase in blood volume through erythropoiesis in utero is adjusted in a chronic fashion, the abrupt increase in blood volume postnatally will be compensated by hemoconcentration resulting in transudation of fluid from the intravascular compartment into the

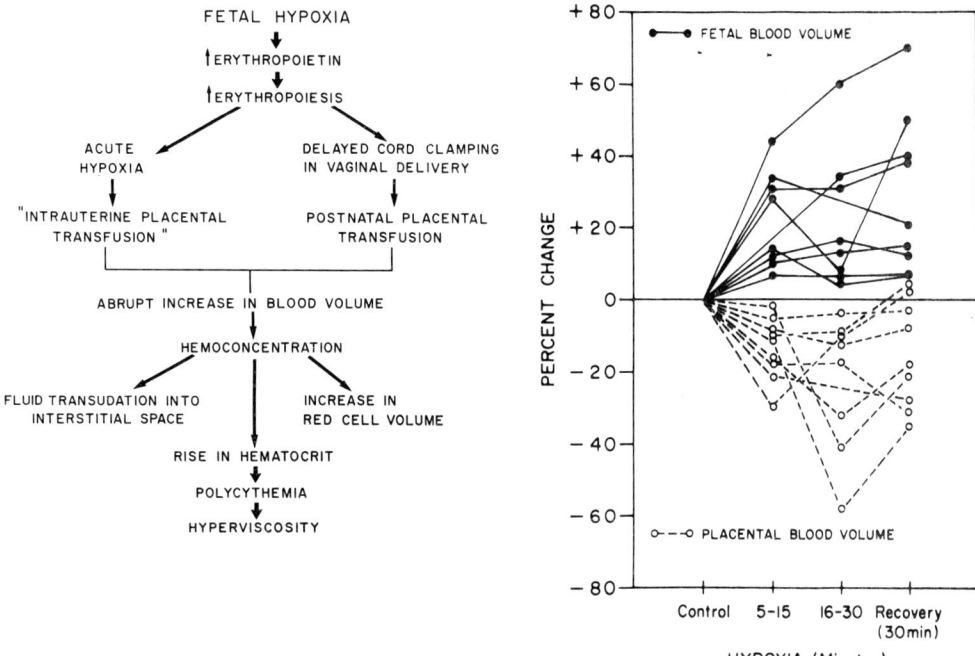

Figure 1. Proposed pathophysiologic role of fetal blood volume changes and neonatal polycythemia and hyperviscosity.

Figure 2 Changes in fetal and placental blood volume during acute fetal hypoxia. From Oh & al., 1975, 722:316.

interstitial space and a rise in hematocrit. The red cell volume will remain high as a result of the transfusion process. The hematocrit of some infants may rise to the point that exceeds the 2 standard deviations which will acquire the status of polycythemia and in these infants the majority will have hyperviscosity on the basis of increase in red cell mass. Therefore, the net effects of the physiologic adaptation following acute transfer of blood into the fetus or neonate from the placenta will result in four phenomena that could singly or in combination account for the various symptoms and signs of polycythemia and hyperviscosity syndrome in a newborn:
1) The pathophysiologic consequence of primary events leading to fetal hypoxia
2) Increase in fluid contents in interstitial tissue in the various organs
3) Hemodynamic effects of polycythemia and hyperviscosity
4) The consequence of elevated red cell volume

The role of fluid transudation into interstitial tissue is an important one and there is evidence for this. In the lung, we have shown that the lung compliance and functional residual capacity in term infants who receive placental transfusion are significantly lower than those who did not. The reduction in lung compliance and functional residual capacity are very likely the function of increased fluid retention in the lung as a result of the transudation process in response to increase in blood volume (Oh et al., 1967). In the

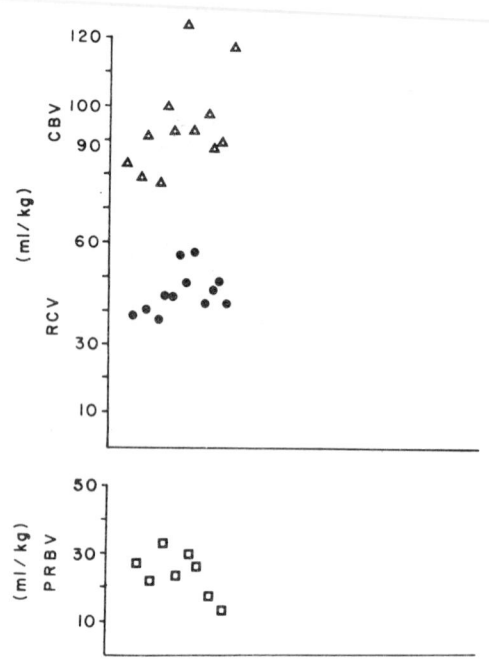

Figure 3. Blood volume (CBV) and red cell blood volume (RCV) in 12 infants delivered vaginally, complicated by perinatal asphyxia and the corresponding placental rise and blood volume (PRBV) in 8 of the 12 infants studied. Umbilical cords were clamped immediately before or a few seconds after birth. Values of normal infants with similar cord clamping time are: CBV 65-70 ml/kg, RCV 31-32 ml/kg, and PRBV 35 ml/kg.

From Yao and Lind 1972, Biol Neonate 21:199-209

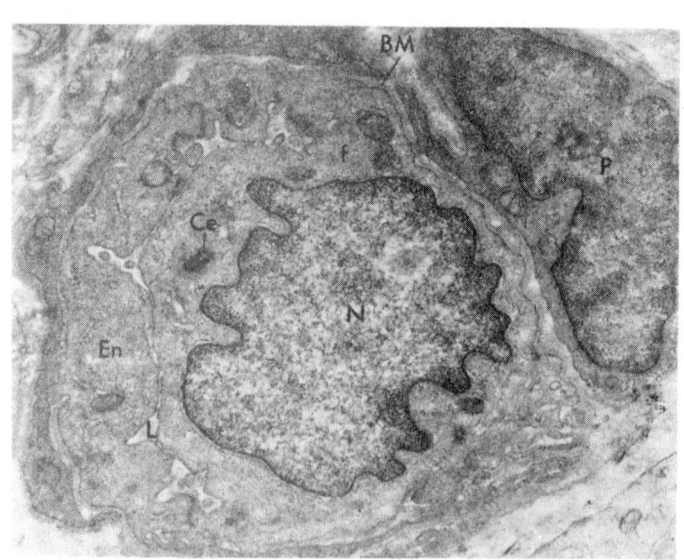

Figure 4. Cutaneous capillary of an infant without placental transfusion. The lumen (L) is reduced to a slit; f, filament; En, endothelial cell; N, nucleus; P, pericyte; Ce, centriole; BM, basement membrane. From: Pietra et al. 1968, Pediatrics 42:678.

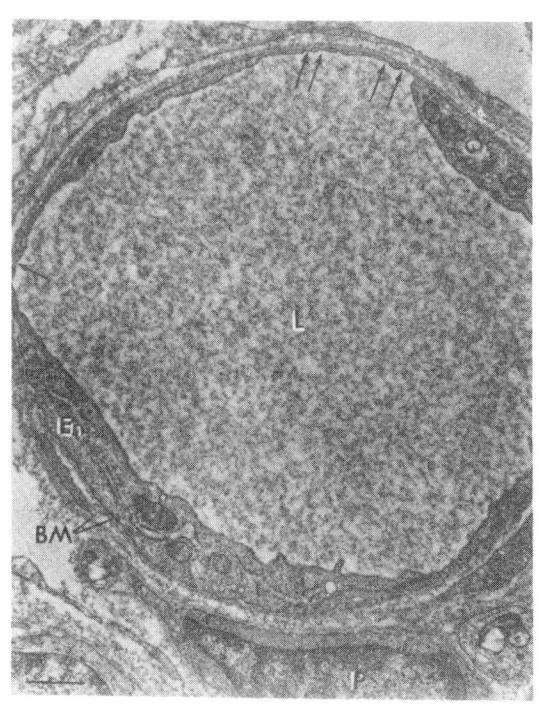

Figure 5. Electronic micrograph of cutaneous capillary of an infant with placental transfusion. Arrows point to fenestrae.

L, lumen; f, filament; En, endothelial cell; N, nucleus; P, pericyte; Ce, centriole; BM, basement membrane.

From: Pietra et al. 1968; Pediatrics 42:678.

skin, we have also demonstrated a significant difference in the cutaneous capillary bed as shown in Figures 4 and 5. In infants who did not receive placental transfusion as a result of early cord clamping, the capillary appeared collapsed, the lumen was reduced to a slit (Figure 4). In contrast, the capillary of the infants with placental transfusion, as shown in figure 5, are markedly distended and show numerous fenestrae which may represent the sites of increased fluid transudation into the extravascular space (Pietra et al., 1968).

CLINICAL PATHOLOGIC CORRELATIONS

It is well known that the symptom complex of polycythemia and hyperviscosity in the newborn are multiorgan and non-specific in nature. The table shows the proposed scheme of how the four factors arising from physiologic changes in response to blood volume alterations can account for the various symptoms that have been described in infants with neonatal polycythemia and hyperviscosity. The signs of jitteriness, tremors, and even seizures, are well known to be associated with sequelae of perinatal asphyxia. Whether fluid transudation and hyperviscosity play a role in producing these symptoms or not is unknown. Cerebral thrombosis has been reported in conjunction with neonatal polycythemia; again, the etiologic explanation of this association is unclear. There is a possibility that in extreme cases of hyperviscosity state, the sludging of flow may be such that it will begin to produce thrombotic phenomenon in cerebral circulation. We have previously indicated that respiratory distress has been associated with neonatal polycythemia and persistent fetal circulation has also been reported. Both can be sequelae of perinatal asphyxia and the respiratory distress can be

Table. Proposed relationship between various events and symptom complex of infants with polycythemia and hyperviscosity.

EVENTS

Organ Related Symptom Complex	Perinatal Asphyxia	Fluid Transudation	Increased Red Cell Mass	Hyperviscosity
CNS				
a) Jitteriness, tremor, seizure	(+)	?	-	?
b) Cerebral Thrombosis	-	-	±	±
Pulmonary				
a) Respiratory Distress	(+)	(+)	-	?
b) Persistent Fetal Circulation	(+)	-	-	?
Heart				
Congestive Heart Failure	±	-	-	?
Gastrointestinal				
a) Feeding Intolerance	(+)	?	-	±
b) Necrotizing Enterocolitis	(+)	?	-	±
Genito-urinary				
Renal Vein Thrombosis	±	-	-	±
Other				
a) Hypoglycemia	(+)	-	±	-
b) Hyperbilirubinemia	-	-	(+)	-

Legend: (+) Very likely association
± Possible association
- Most likely no association
? Unknown

accounted for partly by increased fluid volume in the lung as a result of fluid transudation. The role of hyperviscosity in these two manifestations is also unknown. Acute congestive heart failure has also been reported in infants with polycythemia and hyperviscosity and the etiology is unknown (Michael and Mauer, 1961; Minkowski, 1962 1962). Feeding intolerance and more serious complications in the form of necrotizing enterocolitis has been associated with neonatal polycythemia and hyperviscosity (Hakanson and Oh, 1977; Leblanc et al. 1984; Black et al., in press). Infants with asphyxia are more prone to necrotizing enterocolitis; the exact contribution of the hyperviscosity as well as fluid transudation in regard to gastrointestinal perfusion and oxygenation may contribute to the development of these symptoms but the precise nature of the involvement is still unknown. Renal vein thrombosis has been reported in neonatal polycythemia, and that acute renal failure is also a complication associated with polycythemia in the neonate (Herson et al. 1982). Other potential complications associated with polycythemia and hyperviscosity are: hypoglycemia (Leake et al. 1980; Creswell et al. 1981), and hyperbilirubinemia (Saigal and Usher, 1977). Hypoglycemia is certainly an associated complication of perinatal asphyxia; in addition, the increase in red cell mass may also contribute to the disturbance in glucose homeostasis by an increment in glucose disposal. Erythrocytes are known to be active glycolytic cells in a newborn so that an increase in their number could potentially increase the glucose utilization. The increase in the breakdown of red cells during the first few days of life may also contribute to the increase in bilirubin production resulting in a higher incidence of hyperbilirubinemia in the first few days of life.

REFERENCES

Amit, M., Camfield, P.R. (1980): Neonatal polycythemia causing multiple cerebral infarcts. Arch Neurol 37:109.

Black, V.D., Rumack, C.M., Lubchenco, L.O., Koops, B.L.: Gastrointestinal injury in polycythemic term infants. Pediatrics (in press 1985)

Creswell, J.S., Warburton, D., Susa, J.B., Cowett, R.M., Oh, W. (1981): Hyperviscosity in the newborn lamb produces perturbation in glucose homeostasis. Pediatr Res 15:1348

Finne P.H. (1966): Erythropoietin levels in cord blood as an indicator of intrauterine hypoxia. Acta Paediatr Scand 55:478-489.

Flod, N.E., Ackerman, B.D. (1971): Perinatal asphyxia and residual placental blood volume. Acta Paediatr Scand 60:433-436.

Hakanson, D.O., Oh, W. (1977): Necrotizing enterocolitis and hyperviscosity in the newborn infant. J Pediatr 90:458-461.

Herson, V.C., Raye, J.R., Rowe, J.C., Philipps, A.F. (1982): Acute renal failure associated with polycythemia in a neonate. J Pediatr 100:137

Leake, R.D., Chan, G.M., Zakauddin, S., Dodge, M.E., Fisher, R.H., Bier, O.M., Oh, W. (1980): Glucose perturbation in experimental hyperviscosity. Pediatr Res 14:1320

LeBlanc, M.H., D'Cruz, C., Pate, K. (1984): Necrotizing enterocolitis can be caused by polycythemic hyperviscosity in the newborn dog. J Pediatr 105:804-809.

Michael, A.F., Mauer, A.M. (1961): Maternal-fetal transfusion as a cause of plethora in the neonatal period. Pediatrics 28:458

Minkowski, A. (1962): Acute cardiac failure in connection with neonatal polycythemia (in monovular twins and single newborn infants). Biol Neonate 4:61-74

Oh, W., Wallgren, G., Hanson, J.S., Lind, J. (1967): The effects of placental transfusion on respiratory mechanics of normal term newborn infants. Pediatrics 40:6-12.

Oh, W., Omori, K., Emmanouilides, G.C., Phelps, D.L. (1975): Placenta to lamb fetus transfusion in utero during acute hypoxia. Amer J Obstet Gynecol 122:316-322

Philip, A.G.S., Yee, A.B., Rosy, M., Surti, N., Tsamtsouris, A., Ingall, D. (1969): Placental transfusion as an intrauterine phenomenon in deliveries complicated by fetal distress. Brit Med J. 2:11

Pietra,G.G., D'Amodio,M.D., Leventhal,M.M., Oh,W., Braudo,J.L.(1968): Electron microscopy of cutaneous capillaries of newborn infants: effects of placental transfusion. Pediatrics 42:678-683.

Saigal,S., Usher,R.H.(1977):Symptomatic neonatal plethora. Biol Neonate 32:62-72.

Stevens, K., Wirth,F.H.(1980): Incidence of neonatal hyperviscosity at sea level. J Pediatr 97:118-119

Widness,J.A.,Susa,J.B.,Garcia,J.F., Singer,D.B., Sehgal,P., Oh,W., Schwartz,R., Schwartz,H.C.(1981): Increased erythropoiesis and elevated erythropoietin in infants born to diabetic mothers and in hyperinsulinic Rhesus fetuses. J Clin Invest 67:637-642.

Wirth,F.H., Goldberg,K.E., Lubchenco,L.O.(1979): Neonatal hyperviscosity:I.Incidence.Pediatrics 63:833

Yao,A.C., Lind,J.(1972): Blood volume in the asphyxiated neonate. Biol Neonate 21:199-209.

Yao,A.C., Lind,J.(1982): Placental Transfusion, A Clinical and Physiological Study, Springfield Ill.:Charles C.Thomas Publ.

RESUME.

La polycythemie et l'hyperviscosité constituent des problèmes fréquents de la période néonatale (2,7 à 5%). Le volume sanguin de l'unité foeto-placentaire se répartit pour deux tiers dans le foetus et pour un tiers dans le placenta. Une redistribution de ce volume en faveur du foetus produit une expansion du volume sanguin fetal; une telle redistribution a lieu à la naissance en cas de clampage tardif du cordon et elle exige une adaptation physiologique de la part du nouveau-né (déplacement liquidien transcapillaire vers l'espace extra-cellulaire avec élévation de l'hématocrite). La figure 1 présente les mécanismes physiopathologiques mis en jeu par les modifications du volume sanguin foetal, et la polycythémie et l'hyperviscosité néonatales. L'hypoxie foetale chronique peut entrainer une augmentation du volume sanguin foeto-placentaire par le biais d'une érythropoièse accrue sous l'eefet de l'élévation réactionnelle de l'érythropoïétine. Pendant le travail, l'hypoxie foetale aigue entraine une redistribution brutale du volume sanguin placentaire vers le la circulation foetale. Enfin, la transfusion placentaire néonatale est bien connue. Des altérations cliniques plus ou moins liées à la polycythémie et à l'hyperviscosité sanguine sont résumées dans la Table (essentiellement des perturbations respiratoires, parfois une insuffisance cardiaque, peut-être l'entérite ulcéro-nécrosante,des altérations rénales, une hypoglycémie, et une hyperbilirubinémie).

****

DISCUSSION. Pr.P.Karlberg moderator.

Dr.J.Metcoff: Why do you use a blood volume of 85 ml/kg to correct polycythemia rather than 100 ml/kg? Secondly, the mechanism of placental transfusion does not rely only on stripping the cord or delay in clamping the cord: we have instances of polycythemia when new rotating obstetric housestaff deliver babies and they hold the baby 18 to 27 centimeters below the perineum!

Dr W.Oh: In regard to your second point, the position of the baby at birth certainly makes a difference; 10 centimeters difference between the perineaum and the infant is enough to get a placental transfusion. The gradient is between the infant's right atrial pressure and placental vascular pressure. I don't know whether further down will produce more placental transfusion, probably so but not so very much because at a ceratin point the placental transfusion will begin to level off. As to the formula, 100 or 85 ml/kg body weight as blood volume probably makes very little difference. The real issue is whether you should exchange-transfuse the baby or not, and there is no absolute answer.

Dr. J. Metcoff: Occasionally, we increase the volume of body fluid by therapy with intravenous saline solutions in these babies, which will frequently reduce the hematocrit. Do you think this maneuver might be harmful? Perhaps we are increasing the transudation into the pulmonary alveoli and lymph.

Dr. W. Oh: First of all, I don't really think that increasing fluid intake will necessarily lower the hematocrit. Secondly, there is a potential risk of fluid overload if excessive amount of fluid is given to an infant who has a relatively low renal functional reserve.

Dr. J. Warshaw: Is the position of the baby really an issue? Are there any data showing that the position really contributes to placental transfusion?

Dr. W. Oh: The blood volume in a baby will depend a lot on the level of the infant relative to the perineum. Some of the mother-infant bonding enthusiasts put the baby on the mother's abdomen, and the cord is left dangling: this situation often leads to hypovolemia.

Dr. A. Yao: We found that when we lowered the baby by about 40 cms, the placental transfusion could be completed within 30 seconds. Conversely, elevating the baby above placental level, we found graded decreases in the amount of placental transfusion, depending on the height and the negative pressure gradient created against uteroplacental pressure before cord clamping (Lancet 1969 II: 505). One could abolish placental transfusion or produce hypovolemia by elevating the baby and hypervolemia by lowering the baby

Dr. B. Friis-Hansen: More and more data are accumulating which indicate that cesarean-section protects small premature infants against intraventricualr haemorrhage However, when the baby is taken out by C-section, usually the cord is clamped immediately, which prevents placental transfusion Do you think this is beneficial or should it be avoided? Some people, e.g. Peter Dunn in England, advocates that the cord should not be clamped immediately, and that the baby and the placenta should be taken out at the same time and placed side by side allowing time for lung expansion and a balanced placental transfusion before the cord is clamped. What is your opinion?

Dr. W. Oh: The issue of C-section and premature infants with RDS needs clarification. From all the published series, there is evidence that elective C-section may increase the severity of RDS because of a tendency of increased lung fluid as a result of C-section delivery. In regard to blood volume and RDS, there is no hard evidence that the two are related. In the sixties, Dr. Usher showed RDS premature infants who had lower blood volumes had poorer outcome. However the blood volume determinations were done at 24-48 hours of age and there were no initial determinations of blood volumes Thus one cannot be sure whether there is a cause-effect relationship between blood volume and RDS.

Dr.R.Arcilla: I would like to raise a question concerning blood volume determinations in the newborn period as well as in severely asphyxiated subjects. It pertains to the basic principle or assumption that the plasma concentration of the indicator can be utilized to estimate its volume of distribution, i.e., in the intravascular compartment. One has to assume that the indicator substance distributes itself readily in the various compartments of the circulation and, more importantly, remains within the vascular compartment. I wonder whether increased vascular permeability which promotes transudation of plasma and, possibly, of the indicator substance as well, could result in falsely high blood volume estimations. Could the so-called hypervolemia following birth asphyxia be explained by this mechanism?

Dr.W.Oh: This is a very good question and your concern regarding the potential error introduced by the extravascular leak of the indicator during plasma volume determination is a valid one. In the normal infants, this probably will not occur. However, there is certainly the potential possibility of the increase in capillary permeability which may promote leak of the indicator, giving rise to a falsely high plasma volume. Whether this occurs in the studies in which blood volume was determined following birth asphyxia is not known. On the other hand, a decrease in placental residual blood volume was found to be associated with infants who have asphyxia at birth. If the reciprocal increase in neonatal blood volume is assumed, the findings would support the concept that hypervolemia is indeed present in infants following birth asphyxia.

Dr.G.Moriette: You showed the results of an experimental study by Rosenkrantz et al.(J Pediatr 1984, 104:276) in the newborn lamb in which the oxygen delivery to the brain was maintained constant in spite of hyperviscosity and a reduction of cerebral blood flow. Other data by Leblanc et al.(J Pediatr 1984, 105:804) suggest that polycythemic hyperviscosity in the newborn dog can cause necrotizing enterocolitis (NEC). These results look a bit conflicting, or are the mechanisms or effects different?

Dr.W.Oh: They are not conflicting. On the one hand, Dr.Rosenkrantz' paper refers to the blood flow to the brain while Leblanc's paper deals with blood flow changes to the GI tract. It is well known that under adverse conditions such as hypoxia or polycythemia, the circulatory compensation is different in various organs: brain is more likely to be preferentially protected at the expense of other organs of lower priority such as the GI tract. Therefore, these apparently conflicting results may be explained on the basis of different circulatory adjustments under polycythemic and hyperviscous conditions

Dr.L.Stern: Is there any information on how long a period of asphyxia should be or at what point in gestation should it occur before polycythemia is induced?

Dr.W.Oh: No, not to my knowledge

Neonatal peripheral circulation
Circulation périphérique chez le nouveau-né

Cerebral blood flow in the newborn infant

B. Friis-Hansen

Department of Neonatology, University Hospital, Rigshospitalet, Copenhagen, Denmark

ABSTRACT

Brain injury in preterm infants is one of the most important problems in todays perinatal medicine, as about 7 per cent of all preterm infants develop germinal matrix-intraventricular hemorrhage or hypoxic - ischemic encephalopathy. In this connection the measurement of cerebral blood flow plays a key role. In the following paper various methods for measuring cerebral blood flow is discussed and some of the results obtained will be presented.1)

KEY WORDS

Cerebral blood flow, premature infants, intraventricular hemorrhage

INTRODUCTION

For us who got our education during the war, when very little research was carried out, Johny Lind became our great source of inspiration, when we were able to go to Sweden after the war. His help and keen interest and stimulation has been of tremendous value for the development of Danish pediatric research.

A Danish philosopher once said, "If you want fame for your name, choose something simple and make it complicated". Johny did exactly the opposite, he attacked complicated problems, analysed them by experiments and presented results of outstanding clinical importance in simple terms, which everyone could understand.

In my paper about cerebral blood flow (CBF) in the neonatal period, I shall start by giving a short survey of the various methods available for measuring CBF, and then discuss some of the results obtained. Some of these results are confusing and even such fundamental parameters as normal values for cerebral blood flow in the newborn period, is still not known. Also the role of changes in CBF in the development of germinal matrix-intraventricular hemorrhage (IVH) and hypoxic-ischemic encephalopathy in newborn infants of very low birth weight is also an open question e.g. is low CBF causing IVH or the result of a lesion already present?

We started to measure changes in CBF in newborn infants some ten years ago (Lou, 1977, Lou 1979b) as we felt that CBF was an important factor in the development of

1) The work described here was carried out in collaboration with Hans Lou, Gorm Greisen and other members of the staff.

IVH, a complication, which just had been demonstrated in up to fifty per cent of newborn premature infants with a birth weight below 15oo g.

SUBJECTS AND METHODS

The blood supply to the brain
First a few words about the blood supply to the brain. The main supply of arterial blood is by the internal carotid arteries, which inside the skull split into the anterior and the median cerebral arteries. A smaller, but varying part of the blood is supplied by the vertebral arteries, which fuse to form the basal artery, which devide into the two posterior cerebral arteries, which by the posterior communicating arteries are connected with the two anterior cerebral arteries, which again are connected by the anterior communicating artery. This system of communicating arteries forms the circulus arteriosus of Willi. The external carotid arteries supply all extra cranial tissues of the head and face.

The venous drainage from the brain includes two systems, one superficial set of veins on the surface of the brain, which mainly takes the blood from the cortex and a system of deeper veins, which mainly drains the blood from the deeper regions of the brain, and partly follow the arterial system. Both sets of veins communicate by various plexus and enter the venous sinuses and finally empty into the internal jugular veins.

Thus it is evident that it is not possible to obtain exact values of either total or regional cerebral blood flow by measuring the flow of any single artery or vein.

Methods for measuring CBF in newborn infants
In "Table 1" are listed some of the methods which have been used for measuring CBF in the newborn infant and the year they are introduced. Some methods give absolute values, and some only relative values.

Table 1. Methods for measuring CBF in newborn infants

ABSOLUTE VALUES

KETY-SCHMIDT, N_2O A-V DIFF.	1954
VENOUS OCCLUSION PLETHYSMOGRAPHY	1976
Xe-133 (i.a./i.v./inhal.)	1977

RELATIVE VALUES

ULTRASONIC-DOPPLER TECHNIQUE (FLOW VELOCITY)	1979
ELECTRICAL IMPEDANCE (PULSE VOLUME)	1981
PET SCAN (METABOLISM)	1983
NMR (METABOLISM)	1984

The Kety-Schmidt Method

The Kety-Schmidt method was first used in infants and children in 1953 by Baird and Garfunkel and later in 1957 by Kennedy and Sokoloff, and in 1976 by Settergren. This method is based upon the Fick principle whereby the flow to an organ can be determined from the disappearance rate of a tracer substance (e.g. N_2O) which after injection or inhalation has been distributed evenly in the organ in question. This requires the measurement of the arterial - venous difference during the disappearance period, but in order to measure CBF, certain assumptions must be made. First the tracer substance should not be metabolised during the period of observation. Secondly the distribution should be even, and third the partition coefficient between blood and brain tissue should be known - and should not change during the experiment or vary from person to person. Finally the tracer should diffuse freely so that diffusion is not a rate limiting factor.

The limitation for its use in infants is of course that simultaneous arterial and venous blood samples usually only can be taken in infants during anaesthesia e.g. under operations.

The Xenon Method

The Xenon method is also based upon the Fick principle and in adults this method is considered the standard method for measuring CBF (Hoedt-Rasmussen, 1966). In 1978 it was introduced by Hans Lou and myself to measure CBF in distressed newborn infants. By this method the disappearance rate from the brain is measured after the injection of minute amounts of Xe-133. This is a radioactive gamma-ray emitting isotope with a short half life of 5.2 days. It can either be inhaled as a gas or injected dissolved in saline. In adults the best results are obtained by injecting the Xenon into the internal carotid artery and during the first circulation, Xenon will be distributed in the brain and some of the activity is carried away by the veins. This activity goes directly to the lungs, where practically all is exhaled during the first circulation. No residual activity will therefore be carried back to the brain. The slope of the disappearance curve is therefore a direct measure of cerebral blood flow, when the partition coefficient between the blood and the brain tissue is known.

As injection into the carotid artery of the newborn infant, only can be carried out under special conditions, we have later adapted the intravenous method.

After intravenous injection of Xenon, the activity is first carried to the lungs, where the fraction is exhaled. Then the rest will be distributed evenly over the whole body. After rapid equilibration it is being mobilized again from the tissues and goes back into circulation. Therefore the arterial blood to the brain during the observation period will carry some activity due to re-circulation. The cerebral clearance curve must therefore be corrected for this input, which can be estimated by placing a collimated crystal scintillation detector over the right side of the chest, assuming that the activity in alveolar blood equals that of the arterial blood allowing a delay of 2 sec due to circulation time. By placing a scintillation detector over the head the cranial clearance curve can be measured and by feeding the results of both alveolar and cranial activity into a computer, the disappearance curve can be deconvoluted and flow calculated. The different curves obtained are shown in "Fig. 1" and it is seen that the corrected curve presents at least 2 slopes: An early, fast rate followed by a second, somewhat slower rate.

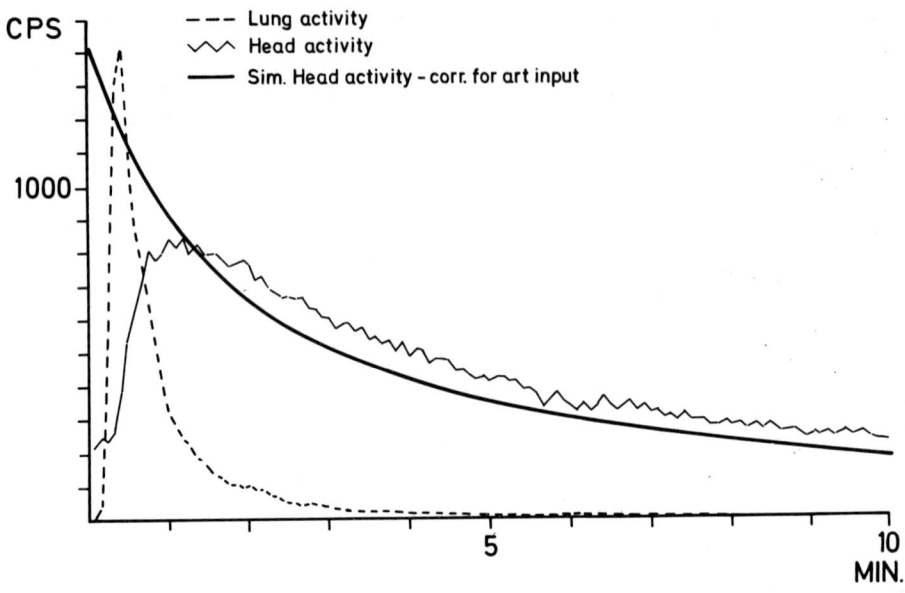

Figure 1. A computer corrected cranial clearance curve and the activity over the right lung after i.v. injection of Xe-133 in a newborn infant (Friis-Hansen, 1985a)

In adults the fast rate is taken to express grey matter flow, and the second, slower slope is regarded as representing white matter flow. In infants such clear cut distinctions cannot be made, partly due to the relatively poor development of the grey matter in the premature brain.

We believe therefore, that the flow measured from 1 to 11 minutes after injection is the best measure of the total cerebral blood flow (Greisen, 1984), although the values calculated this way are only about 2/3 of those reported earlier (Lou, 1977, Friis-Hansen, 1979a). Therefore, unfortunately, each measurement takes about 15 minutes, and brief changes in CBF cannot be detected. Furthermore, although the radiation dose for one measurement is very low, corresponding to only about 1/10 of a chest X-ray, this sets a limit for how many times the examination can be repeated, but with all these limitations this method still is supposed to give the most reliable figures for cerebral blood in absolute figures. The i.v. Xe-133 method has also been used in preterm infants by Younkin (1982), but he used the same partition coefficient between grey- and white matter and blood as for adults (0.85 and 1.5) whereas we have found the coefficients to be only 0.85 and 0.85 in the newborn infants (Greisen, 1984). These coefficients will reduce the total flow with up to one third.

In adults Xe-133 may also be administred by inhalation from a closed system. This method was tried by Ment in 1981, in very small premature infants, but the technical difficulties and errors are greater than by the i.a. or i.v. administration.

The Doppler Technique

The ultrasonic Doppler technique has recently been used extensively in newborn infants. It is harmless, quick, and can be repeated with intervals of only seconds. It has therefore been used widely, although it measures only flow velocities and not volumes. The principle and a typical curve is showed in "Fig. 2". Ultrasound waves are generated and send as a narrow band against the vessels studied, and according to the Doppler principle, the frequency of the reflected waves will shift depending on the velocity and direction of the blood flow in question. "Fig. 2".

Measurement of blood flow velocity by doppler ultrasound

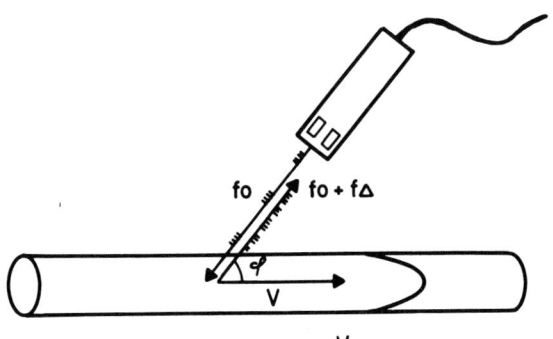

$$\Delta f = 2 \cdot f_o \cdot \cos\varphi \cdot \frac{V}{C}$$

C = vel. of sound in tissue

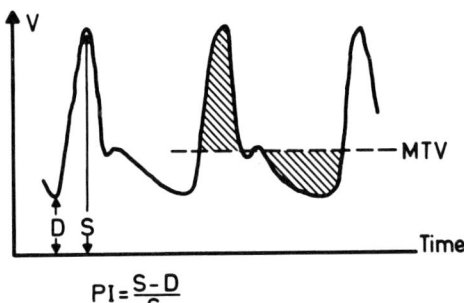

$$PI = \frac{S-D}{S}$$

Figure 2. Measurement of arterial CBF by ultrasound, using the Doppler principle. Fo is the original sound frequency. Δf is the frequency change. Ø is the angle to the vessel. V is the velocity of the blood and C is the velocity of ultrasound in tissue. D is the diastolic velocity, S the peak systolic velocity and MFV the mean flow velocity. PI is the pulsatility index. (Friis-Hansen, 1985b).

Different parts of the curve can be used to estimate flow, either the "systolic peak flow velocity","the diastolic flow velocity", "the mean flow velocity", "the pulsatility index", as discussed by Volpe (1982). All these parameters are expression of flow velocity and changes in flow velocity. It is, however, easily understood, that changes in peripheral resistance can give higher amplitudes and changes in the caliber of the vessel can give changes in flow velocity, but without changes in flow volume. Yet the method is easy and can be repeated at short intervals, and it has been used widely to study changes in flow rates related to age and various physiological and pathological conditions. We tried to compare the Doppler technique to the Xe-133 method and found a relatively poor correlation in the human infant (Greisen, 1984). In animals others have found a better correlation (Hansen, 1983).

The Venous Occlusion Plethysmographic Method

The venous occlusion plethysmographic method was introduced by Cross and his collaborators in 1976. The elegant principle of this method is based upon the assumption that minute increases in cranial volume can be detected, when the venous outflow suddenly is stopped by compressing the jugular vein for a few seconds. This increase in volume is a measure of cerebral blood flow if in-flow remains unchanged. The changes in cranial volume can be calculated by measuring the increase in the occipitofrontal circumference by a strain gauge.

The underlying principle is that the cranium is freely expansible and that the soft tissue outside the brain only gives a minor error. The rate of increase is a measure of cerebral blood flow, assuming that dilation of the cranium is equal in all directions, but unfortunately this does not seem to be the case (Cooke, 1977).

Cerebral electrical impedance

A method has also been developed to measure CBF in newborn infants by placing two sets of electrodes over the head and measure the changes in electrical impedance which takes place during each pulse-stroke, or by measuring changes in a weak constant electrical current. These changes seem to follow the stroke volume, but the actual calibration may be difficult and comparison with the vascular occlusion plethysmography showed poor reproduceability (Reigel, 1977, Costeloe, 1984).

The PET Scanning and the NMR Scanning

The PET scanning (Volpe, 1983) and the NMR (nuclear magnetic resonance) scanning (Hope, 1984) measure the rate of metabolism in various regions of the brain and thereby indirectly blood flow, but these methods do not give any absolute values for cerebral blood flow.

Before discussing some of the results obtained in newborn infants by these methods, I would like to point out a few facts about CBF in the dog, where it has been studied extensively. The grey matter flow is 2-3 times higher than that of the white matter, and in both groups the grey matter flow is very sensitive to variations in both arterial carbondioxide tension. Furthermore in normal adult dogs, CBF is about twice as high as that found in puppies (Shapiro, 1980), and finally CBF is almost constant over a wide range of variation in blood pressure. In puppies this range extends from 4o to 8o mmHg and in the adult dog from 6o to 1oo mmHg. Below these pressure limits, CBF decreases, and above CBF increases. Similar results have been obtained in other species, including the human adult and newborn babies (Lou, 1979a, Lou, 1979b). "Fig. 3".

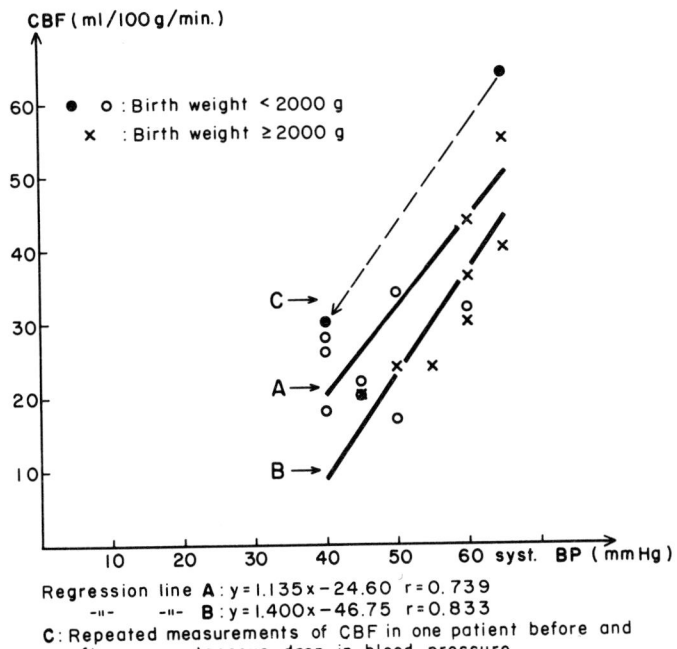

Figure 3. Pressure passive CBF in distressed newborn infants (Lou, 1979a)

This ability of the brain to maintain a constant flow during variations in blood pressure demonstrates autoregulation of CBF and it protects the brain by maintaining a constant internal milieu in spite of fluctuations in blood pressure and blood gasses. Shortly it may be said that CBF is tailored to meet the need of cerebral metabolism (Tweed, 1983).

This autoregulation is presumably related to the blood-brain barrier and a breakdown - reversible or irreversible - of autoregulation by changes in parameters such as asphyxia, hypercarbia, increased blood pressure, acidosis, hypoglycemia or hyperosmolarity - all factors which have been described as beeing etiological factors in the development of IVH "Fig. 4".

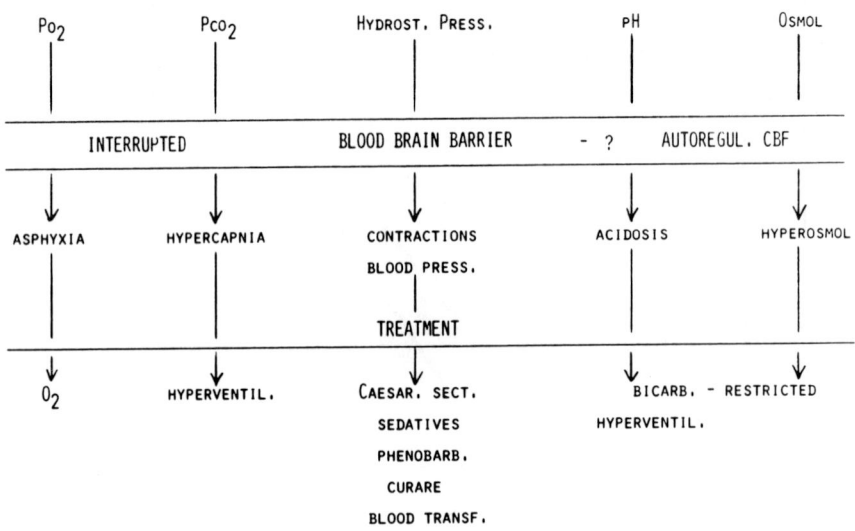

Figure 4. Factors causing a breakdown of the blood brain barrier are presumably also responsible for impairment of autoregulation of CBF (Friis-Hansen, 1985a).

Normal values for CBF in newborn infants
As described above the most acurate measurements of CBF in the newborn human infant have been obtained by the Kety-Schmidt and the Xe-133 methods, but as both are "invasive" hardly any determinations have been carried out in normal full term and mature infants. By the venous occlusion method, which is non-invasive, values in normal full term infants around 4o ml/loo g/min have been found by Cross (1979) and as high as 63 ml/loo g/min by Leahy (1979) and lower values 31 ml/loo g/min have been measured in premature infants (Leahy, 198o).

In adults a CBF of 6o-8o ml/loo g/min by the Xe-133 method is considered normal. The N_2O technique has given highly varying results in sedated infants and children with values from 3o to 1o6 ml/loo g/min (Baird, 1953, Kennedy, 1957, Settergren 1976).

We have studied distressed infants with the Xe-133 method mostly during treatment with assisted ventilation, but a few infants had only minor disturbances and were considered "well", but non were completely "normal".

Our results are summarized in "Fig. 5".

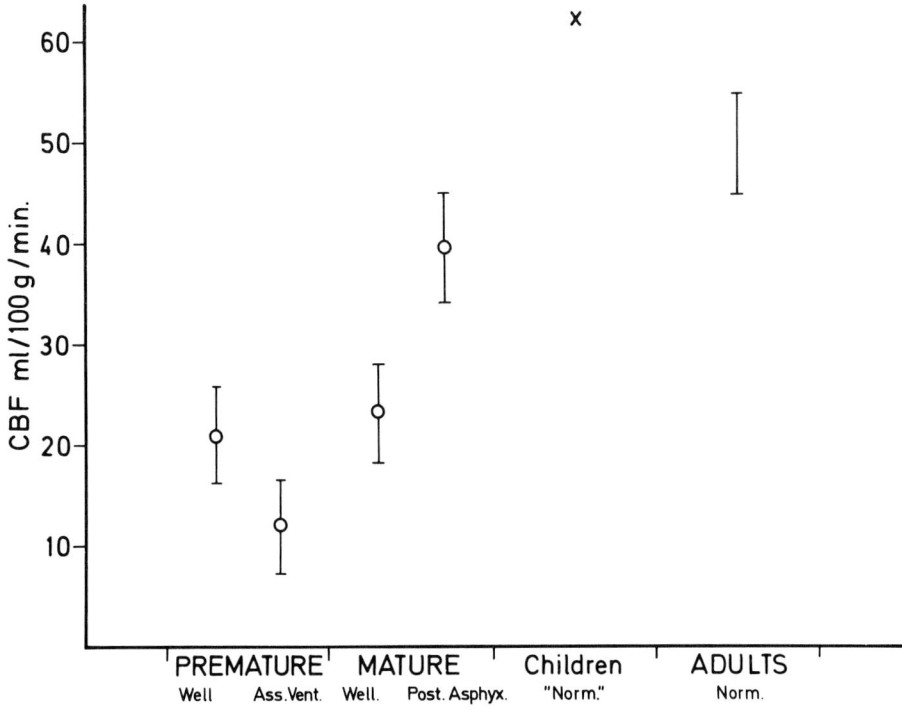

Figure 5. CBF in infants, children and adults (Friis-Hansen, 1985a).

CBF in well premature infants is around 2o ml/1oo g/min. In stressed premature infants treated with assisted ventilation the flow is around 12 ml/1oo g/min. In mature "well" infants the flow is around 23 ml/1oo g/min. In post asphyxiated infants values as high as 4o ml/1oo g/min were found. This may be an example of "the luxury perfusion syndrome". (Lassen, 1966).

In normal children values around 6o ml/1oo g/min have been reported as compared to values around 5o ml/1oo g/min reported in normal adults.

As described above, changes in cerebral blood flow may play a key role in the development of IVH. This is illustrated in "Fig. 6", which shows that impaired autoregulation of CBF gives a pressure passive blood flow thus arterial hypotension will aggrevate any ischemia present, whereas arterial hypertension will increase the risk of bleeding from the capillaries (Friis-Hansen, 1981).

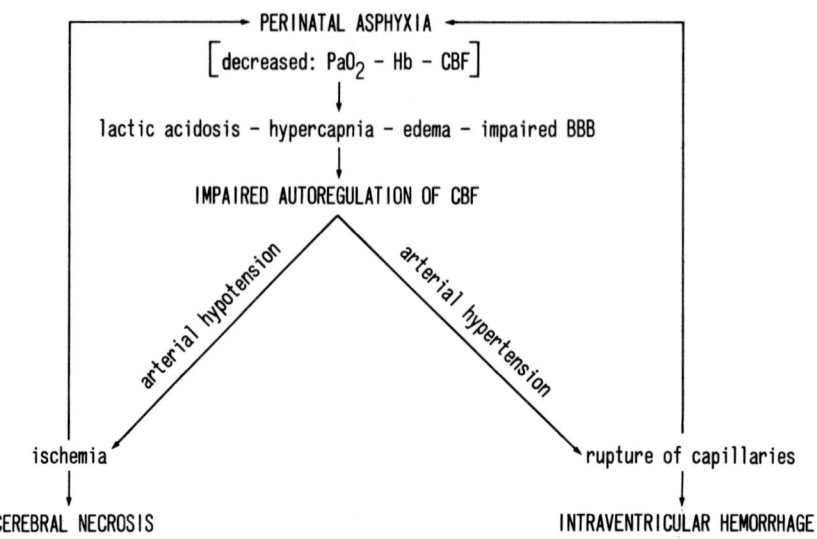

Figure 6. Diagram illustrating the role of impaired autoregulation of CBF in the development of IVH (Friis-Hansen, 1981).

Fluctuations in CBF velocity has been described as an important etiological factor in IVH. Therefore sedation of small premature infants undergoing intensive care has been suggested as a prophylactic measure (Friis-Hansen, 1979). Thus it has been demonstrated recently that muscular paralysis induced by the injection of pancuronium in premature infants with a fluctuating pattern of CBF velocity, protected them against IVH (Perlman, 1985).

REFERENCES

Baird, H.W., Garfunkel, J.M. (1953): A method for the measurement of cerebral blood flow in infants and children. J Pediatr 42, 57o-575.
Costeloe, K., Smyth, D.P., Murdoch, N. et al (1984): A comparison between electrical impedance and strain gauge plethysmography for the study of cerebral blood flow in the newborn. Pediatr Res, 18, 29o-295.
Cooke, R.W.I., Rolfe, R., Eng, C. et al (1977): A technique for the noninvasive estimation of cerebral blood flow in the newborn infant. J Med Eng Technol I, 263-266.
Cross, K.W., Dear, P.R.F., Warner, R.M. et al (1976): An attempt to measure cerebral blood flow in the newborn infant. J Physiol, 26o, 42-43.
Cross, K.W., Dear, P.R.F, Harthorn, M.K.S. et al (1979): An estimate of intracranial blood flow in the newborn infant. J Physiol, 289, 329-345.

Friis-Hansen, B., Lou, H.C., Marstrand-Christiansen, P., Scheibel, E. (1979): The influence of apnea and physical activity on arterial blood pressure and transcutaneous oxygen tension in the newborn. In Continuous transcutaneous blood gas monitoring, eds A. Huch, R. Huch, J.F. Lucey, pp 461-468, New York: Alan R. Liss Inc.

Friis-Hansen, B., Lou, H.C., Lassen, N.A., Wimberley, P.D. (1981): The pathogenesis of cerebral hypoxic lesions and intraventricular hemorrhage in the newborn preterm infant. In Intensive care in the newborn III, eds L Stern, B. Salle, B. Friis-Hansen, pp 253-62, U.S.A.: Masson.

Friis-Hansen, B. (1985a): Perinatal brain injury and cerebral blood flow in newborn infants. Acta Paediatr Scand, 74, 323-331.

Friis-Hansen, B., Greisen, G., Ellison, P.H., Johansen, K.H., Frederiksen, P.S., Mali, J. (1985b): Cerebral blood flow in the newborn: Comparison of two methods of Doppler ultrasound and Xenon 133 clearance, In Physiologic foundations of perinatal medicine, eds S. Stern, M. Xanthou, B. Friis-Hansen, pp.325-333, Praeger.

Greisen, G., Frederiksen, P.S., Mali, J., Friis-Hansen, B. (1984a): Analysis of cranial 133-Xenon clearance in the newborn infant by the two-compartment model. Scand J Clin Lab Invest, 44, 239-25o.

Greisen, G., Johansen, K., Ellison, P.H., Frederiksen, P.S., Mali, J., Friis-Hansen, B. (1984b): Cerebral blood flow in the newborn infant: Comparison of Doppler ultrasound and 133-Xenon clearance. J Pediatr, 1o4, 411-418.

Hansen, N.B., Stonestreet, B.S., Rosenkrantz, T.S., Oh, W. (1983): Validity of Doppler measurements of anterior cerebral artery blood flow velocity: Correlation with brain blood flow in piglets. Pediatrics, 72, 526-531.

Hoedt-Rasmussen, K., Sveinsdottier, E., Lassen, N.A. (1966): Regional cerebral blood flow in man determined by intra-arterial injection of radioactive inert gas. Circ Res, 18, 237-247.

Hope, P.L., Cady, E.B., Tofts et al (1984): Cerebral energy metabolism studied with phosphorus NMR spectroscopy in normal and birth asphyxiated infants. Lancet, I, 366-69.

Kennedy, C., Sokoloff, L. (1957): An adaptation of the nitrous oxide method to the study of the cerebral circulation in children: Normal values for cerebral blood flow and cerebral metabolic rate in childhood. J Clin Invest, 36, 113o-1137.

Lassen, N.A. (1966): The luxury perfusion syndrome and its possible relation to acute metabolic acidosis localised within the brain. Lancet, II, 1113-15.

Leahy, F.A.N., Sankaran, K., Cates, D. et al (1979): Quantitative noninvasive method to measure cerebral blood flow in newborn infants. Pediatrics, 64, 277-282.

Leahy, F.A.N., Cates, D., MacCallum, M. et al (198o): Effects of CO_2 and 1oo% O_2 on cerebral blood flow in preterm infants. J Appl Physiol, 48, 468-72.

Lou, H.C., Lassen, N.A., Friis-Hansen, B. (1977): Low cerebral blood flow in hypotensive perinatal distress. Acta Neurol Scand, 56, 343-352.

Lou, H.C., Lassen, N.A., Friis-Hansen, B. (1979a): Impaired autoregulation of cerebral blood flow in the distressed newborn infant. Pediatrics, 94, 118-21.

Lou, H.C., Lassen, N.A., Tweed, W.A., Johnson, G., Jones, M., Palahniuk, R.J. (1979b): Pressure passive cerebral blood flow and breakdown of the blood-brain barrier in experimental fetal asphyxia. Acta Paediatr Scand, 68, 57-63.

Ment. L.R., Ehrenkranz, R.A., Lange, R.C. et al (1981): Alterations in cerebral blood flow in preterm infants with intraventricular hemorrhage. Pediatrics, 68, 763-769.

Perlman, J.M., Goodman, S., Kreusser, K., Volpe, J.J. (1985): Reduction in intraventricular hemorrhage by elimination of fluctuating cerebral blood flow in preterm infants with respiratory distress syndrome. N Engl J Med, 312, 1353-1387.

Reigel, D.H., Dallman, D.E., Scarff, T.B., Woodford, J. (1977): Transcephalic impedance measurement during infancy. Dev Med Child Neurol, 19, 295-304.
Settergren, G., Linblad, B.S., Persson, B. (1976): Cerebral blood flow and exchange of oxygen, glucose, ketone bodies, lactate, pyruvate and amino acids in infancy. Acta Paediatr Scand, 65, 343-353.
Shapiro, H.M., Greenberg, J.H., Naughton, K.V.H., Reivich, M. (1980): Heterogeneity of local cerebral blood flow-$PaCO_2$ sensitivity in neonatal dogs. J Appl Physiol, 49, 113-118.
Tweed, W.A., Cote, J., Pash, M., Lou, H. (1983): Arterial oxygenation determines autoregulation of cerebral blood flow in the fetal lamb. Pediatr Res, 17, 246.
Volpe, J.J., Perlman, J.M., Hill, A., McMenamin, J.B. (1982): Cerebral blood flow velocity in the human newborn: The value of determination. Pediatrics, 70, 147-150.
Volpe, J.J., Herscovitch, P., Perlman, J.M., Raichle, M.E. (1983): Positron emission tomography in the newborn: Extensive impairment of regional cerebral blood flow with intraventricular hemorrhage and hemorrhagic intracerebral involvement. Pediatrics, 72, 589-601.
Younkin, D.P., Reivich, M., Jaggi, J. et al (1982): Noninvasive method of estimating human newborn regional cerebral blood flow. J Cereb Blood Flow Metab, 2, 415-420.

RESUME.

En médecine néonatale, à l'heure actuelle, les atteintes cérébrales constituent un problème majeur puisque environ 7 pour cent de tous les prématurés présentent une hémorragie de la zone germinative, accompagnée ou non d'une hémorragie intra-ventriculaire (HZG+HIV.) ou une encéphalopathie de type hypoxie-ischémie. Aussi est-il important de disposer de valeurs normales de débit sanguin cérébral chez le nouveau-né, de manière à pouvoir mieux évaluer le rôle de ses altérations dans l'apparition des lésions cérébrales.

Après un rappel de la vascularisation artérielle et du drainage veineux cérébraux, les différentes méthodes de mesure employées par le passé sont brièvement décrites et critiquées. La technique de Kéty-Schmidt basée sur le principe de Fick exigeait des prélèvements artériels et veineux simultanés sous anesthésie et elle n'est plus en usage. La méthode au Xénon 133 a d'abord été utilisée avec l'injection classique de Xenon dans la carotide, et plus tard en recourant à la voie intra-veineuse (l'inhalation de Xe 133 convient aux adultes mais elle entache les résultats de larges erreurs chez le nouveau-né). La technique d'ultrasons à effet Doppler donne surtout des reflets des variations de vélocité du débit. La méthode de pléthysmographie occlusive a été temporairement proposée en 1976-77. La mesure de l'impédance électrique trans-cérébrale note des variations parallèles à celles du volume d'éjection ventriculaire mais la calibration est difficile. Les tomographies en émission de positons ("PET scans") et par résonance magnétique nucléaire (RMN) mesurent le taux du métabolisme dans les diverses régions du cerveau et donc indirectement le débit cérébral, mais sans fournir de chiffres absolus.

Les valeurs normales paraissant les plus exactes ont été obtenues par les méthodes de Kéty-Schmidt et du Xe 133. Les résultats rapportés ici proviennent d'études par le Xe 133 chez des nouveau-nés en détresse, dont certains n'avaient que des perturbations mineures, mais dont aucun n'était "normal".(voir figure 5).

Le schéma 6 montre à quel point les variations passives du débit sanguin cérébral sous l'effet des modifications de pression sanguine, quand l'autorégulation circulatoire cérébrale est altérée, peuvent aggraver l'ischémie cérébrale en phase d'hypotension ou favoriser les saignements capillaires en période d'hypertension. Il est donc suggéré qu'une sédation s'opposant aux fluctuations de vélocité du débit cérébral pourrait avoir un rôle protecteur contre les HZG-HIV.

****

DISCUSSION. Dr.L.Stern moderator.

Dr.H.Lagercrantz: Theophylline decreased cerebral blood flow (CBF). Is it a direct effect or might it be due to a decreased P_{CO_2} ? It is also possible that adenosine might be involved because adenosine has been found to affect CBF.

Pr.B.Friis-Hansen: It seems as if changes in cerebral blood flow are mediated by local changes in the tissue and that vasoactive kinines and prostaglandins in the wall of the blood vessels are responsible for at least a major part of the observed changes. Thus if the P_{CO_2} is increased, changes in CBF will occur almost instantaneously, even before any diffusion of CO2 into the cerebral tissue could have taken place. This indicates that the tonus of the arterioles and capillaries is changing as a result of primary changes taking place in the walls of these vessels as part of the autoregulation of CBF, rather than changes mediated by more distant control mechanisms.

Dr.W.Oh: Rosenkrantz performed Doppler studies (Rosenkrantz & Oh, J Pediatr 1982, 101:94) and recorded cerebral blood flow, velocity in the form of area under the curve (AUTC), in a group of low birth weight infants who received a bolus dose of aminophylline. He found a significant reduction in AUTC which was related primarily to a reduction in P_{CO_2}. Stonestreet et al.(Devel Pharm Therap 1983,6:248) did a similar study in the newborn lamb in whom respiration was controlled (P_{CO_2} remained unchanged), and they found no difference in CBF when aminophyllin was given. Those data suggest that aminophyllin influences CBF primarily through its effect on breathing (hyperpnea lowering the P_{CO_2}).

Dr.B.Lundell: We used a Doppler velocimeter system (Lundell et al, Acta Paediatr Scand 1984, 73:810) to study intracranial hemodynamics in unanesthetized newborn lambs. A single i.v. dose of aminophylline (10 mg /kg) reduced the intracranial blood flow velocities after 15 minutes by 19%. The Pa_{CO_2} fell from 44 to 41 mmHg which should have reduced the blood flow velocity by only 6%. We have therefore some reason to believe that aminophylline reduces CBF by a direct effect on the cerebral circulation rather than via a reduced Pa_{CO_2}.

Pr.P.Karlberg: You recalled the main methods of CBF measurements but you did not comment on PET at the end of the list? We would be grateful for a good monitoring system which could be used over a period of time! And what about the transcephalic impedance?

Pr.B.Friis-Hansen: PET has been used only in a few places (e g Volpe, Pediatrics 1983, 72:589). The basic principle of the lectrical cerebral impedance method is that during each pulsation a certain increase in brain volume will take place, which can be monitored. This method seems to give a good indication of variations in "pressure and flow changes" (see: Weindling et al. Acta Paediatr Scand suppl.311:14, 1983; Ellison et al. Acta Paediatr Scand 1983, 73:820; Mochalova et al. Acta Paediatr Scand suppl 311:20, 1983).

Dr.Ab.Rudolph: Measurements in lambs have shown that brain blood flow is considerably higher during fetal as compared with neonatal life. The fall in brain blood flow after birth is probably the result of the increase in arterial oxygen tension and oxygen content. It has been shown that cerebral oxygen consumption is relatively constant, and that brain blood flow can be modified readily (Jones and Traystman, Sem Perinatol 1984, 8:205), depending on arterial oxygen content. One of the problems with the Doppler technique as you have applied it is that it is not quantitative and the measurements can be affected by many variables.

Pr.B.Friis-Hansen: I fully agree with you that, technically, the methods for measuring regional cerebral blood flow are not refined enough. For example, each measurement by our method takes about 10-15 min. and during that period many changes in flow rates and distribution may have taken place. We have been surprised by the finding of very low flow rates in ventilated small premature infants. Shunting mayhave influenced the Xe133 wash-out curves, but a mathematical model showed that even a shunt of 40 per cent could not account for these very low flow rates.

Dr.Ab.Rudolph: Do you think that PET is going to be the solution to the problem?

Pr.B.Friis-Hansen: PET seems to have a better resolution than the other methods. However, it is more a measurement of energy metabolism than of flow itself.

An animal model for measurements of intracranial blood flow velocities

B.P.W. Lundell, H. Sundell, D.P. Lindstrom and M.T. Stahlman

Departments of Pediatrics, Vanderbilt University, Nashville, TN, USA and Karolinska Institute, Sachs' Children's Hospital, Stockholm, Sweden

SUMMARY

A range-gated Doppler ultrasound velocimeter was used to measure intracranial blood flow velocities via artificial fontanels in newborn lambs. The velocimeter and the computerized analyzing system was thoroughly tested in vitro and in vivo. The technique allows frequent or continuous measurements of intracranial blood flow velocities in unanesthetized animals.
This method may be useful for physiological and farmacological studies of intracranial hemodynamics where invasive techniques could interfere with the results or if the animals can not be sacrificed.

KEY WORDS

Cerebral blood flow, Doppler, animal

INTRODUCTION

Our knowledge about cerebral blood flow and it's regulation in the newborn period is mainly based on animal studies. Methods which are used in infants must be non-invasive and can only provide us with semiquantitative measures of cerebral blood flow (Rolfe, 1984). Invasive techniques, however, can be used in animals for measurements of volume flow. The microsphere technique have been used in most recent studies (Hansen, 1984; Rosenkrantz, 1984). This method allows only a limited number of measurements under a short period of time and the animal must be sacrificed.
Doppler velocimeters have been used in several recent studies of intracranial hemodynamics in newborn infants (Ahman, 1983; Bada, 1979; Gray, 1983; Martin, 1982; Perlman, 1983). However, few have presented any data on the validity of the technique compared to invasive flow measurements (Batton, 1983; Hansen, 1983; Rosenberg, 1985).
The present study was performed in order to validate a range-gated Doppler velocimeter system for use in animal studies. The aim was to test a non-invasiv technique which would permit unlimited number of measurements in unanesthetized newborn animals.

Doppler velocimeter

A combined range-gated and continuous multi-frequency Doppler instrument was used (Alfred, Vingmed A/S, Oslo, Norway). A five MHz transducer with 8 mm crystal diameter was used. All measurements were made in the pulsed mode. The longitudinal sampling interval was set at 2 mm. A high-pass filter with a cut-off frequency at 100 Hz allowed recordings of velocities between 3 and 170 cm per second. The Doppler instrument generated a simulated Doppler shift corresponding to velocities of 0, 10, 20 and 50 cm per second, which were used for calibration of the recordings.

Signal analysis

The maximum and the average Doppler shifts were recorded together with the ECG on a polygraph (HP7758D, Hewlett-Packard, Waltham, MA, USA) and on FM-tape (Vetter Model D, Vetter Co., Rebersburg, PA, USA). The average Doppler shift, over the blood vessels cross section, and the ECG signals were played back and sampled by an analog/digital converter and a PDP 11/34 computer at an effective sampling rate of 250 Hz. The calibration signals were used to compute a linear regression algorithm which was used by the computer program to calculate the velocities. The trailing edge of the ECG signal was used to define each cardiac cycle. A total of 50-100 consecutive beats were averaged. The computer program identified the peak systolic and the end diastolic velocity and calculated the pulsatility index. The average velocity signal was integrated over the sampling period to yield the area under the curve which is the best measure of true flow (Hansen, 1983; Lundell, 1984). A print-out of a computer analyzed average velocity signal is shown in Fig. 1.

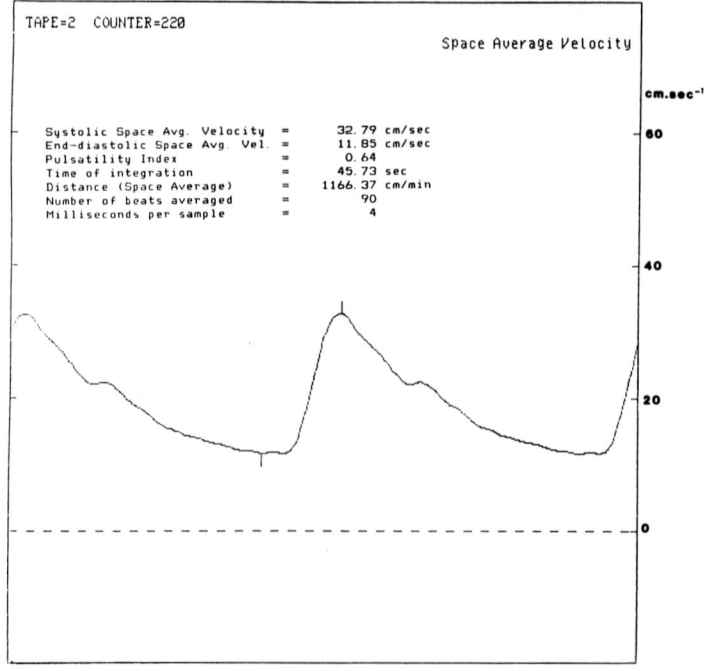

Fig.1. Computer analyzed average velocity recording of 90 consecutive beats. Graphical and numerical presentation of the mean values.

In vitro validation

A pulsatile flow was generated in an in vitro model which is shown in Fig. 2. A continuous flow pump ("venous return") filled a 250 ml plastic bag which was placed on a spring-loaded base. The bag was intermittently compressed by a rotating roller (120 rpm) to generate the pulsatile flow through the artificial blood vessels. Silicon rubber tubings 1.0-2.8 mm in diameter were led through a water-filled box. The Doppler ultrasound beam was directed with a constant angle of 18 degrees towards the tubings. Afterload in the system was changed by elevating the outflow to the measuring glass, where true flow was recorded. The volume flow through the system was varied by changing the flow through the continuous flow pump between 4 and 94 ml/min (Lundell, 1984).

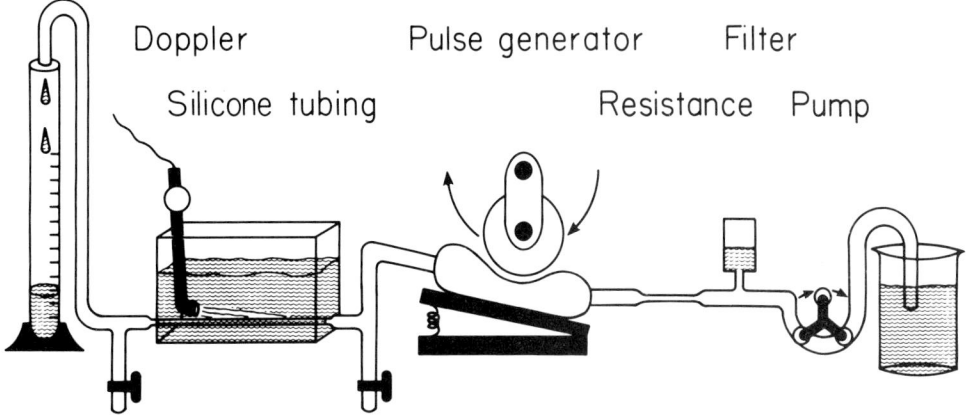

Fig.2. The pulsatile flow model.

The results are summarized in Fig. 3. An excellent correlation was found between true flow and Doppler flow when the average velocity was multiplied by the cross sectional area of the artificial blood vessel. The small negative intercept of the regression line is explained by the 100 Hz wall motion filter which excludes the recording of velocities below 3 cm/sec.

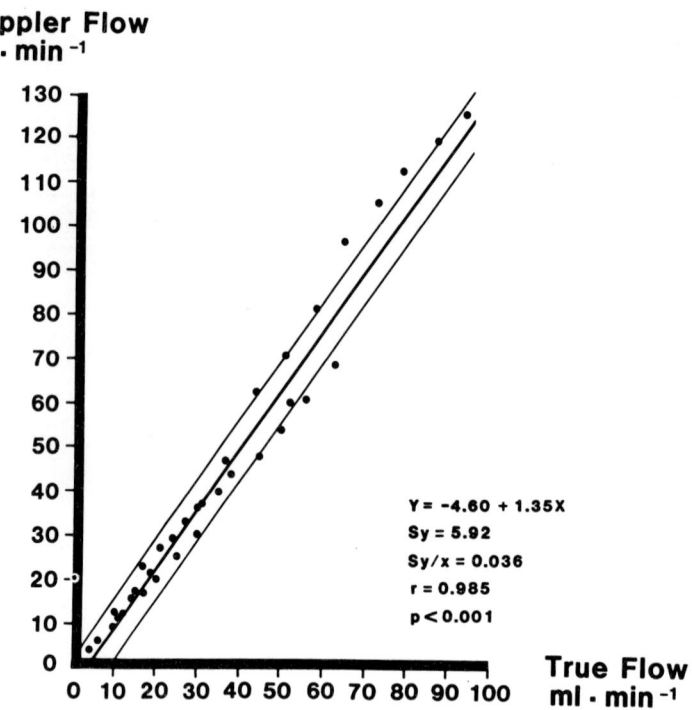

Fig.3. Doppler measured versus true flow in the in vitro model. Regression line and equation.

In vivo validation

Six newborn lambs were studied in acute experiments under general anesthesia. Carotid blood flow on both sides of the neck was measured with 3 mm electromagnetic flow transducers (C&C Instruments, Culver City, CA, USA) which had been calibrated in vitro beforehand using excised blood vessels and saline. Artificial fontanels were made through the skull, close to the midline. The skin-flaps were sutured back and the measurements were made through the skin. The Doppler instrument was switched from continuous to pulsed mode when a strong pulsatile signal was heard and seen on a monitor. The depth setting was increased to the maximum depth where a high arterial flow toward the Doppler probe could still be recorded. This procedure allowed recordings of the Doppler shift in the deepest lying artery which could be found on the intracranial surface of the base of the skull. The mean depth setting used was 3.8 cm (mean body weight:5500 g).

Changes in arterial flow to the head was accomplished by partial or complete occlusions of one or both carotid arteries distal to the flow cuffs. The ECG, blood pressure, carotid blood flow on both sides and the maximum and mean intracranial flow velocity signals were recorded. An example of this is shown in Fig. 4.

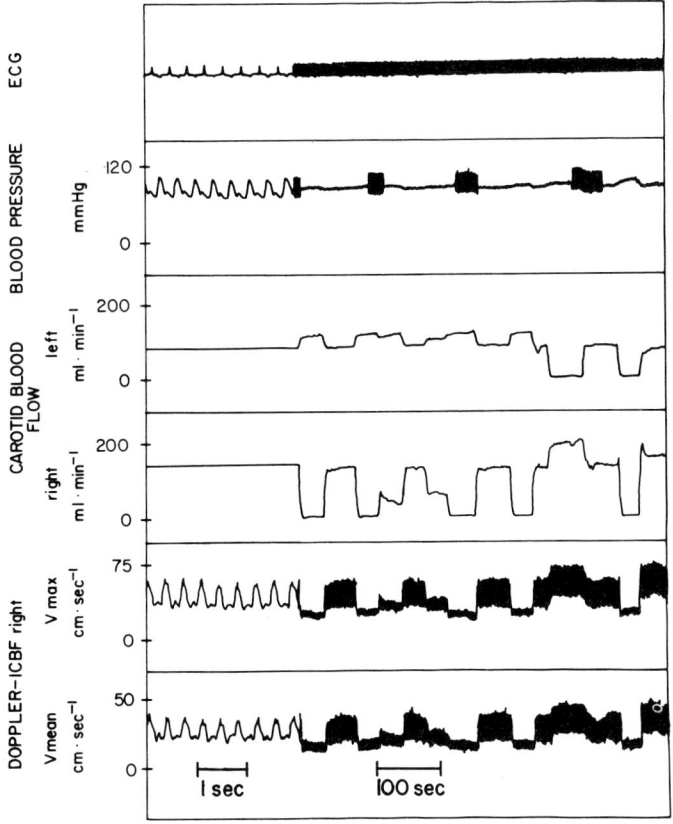

Fig.4. An example of different occlusions of the carotid arteries and the effects on intracranial blood flow velocities. Recordings of electrocardiogram (ECG), arterial blood pressure, carotid blood flow on both sides and intracranial blood flow velocities (Vmax and Vmean) on the right side. Note the congruence between the tracings of right carotid blood flow and the Doppler recordings from the right side in the head.

Measurements were made during at least six different arbitrarily chosen blood flows on each side. Changes in carotid blood flow was compared with the ipsilateral intracranial blood flow velocity. A close correlation was found which is shown in Fig. 5.

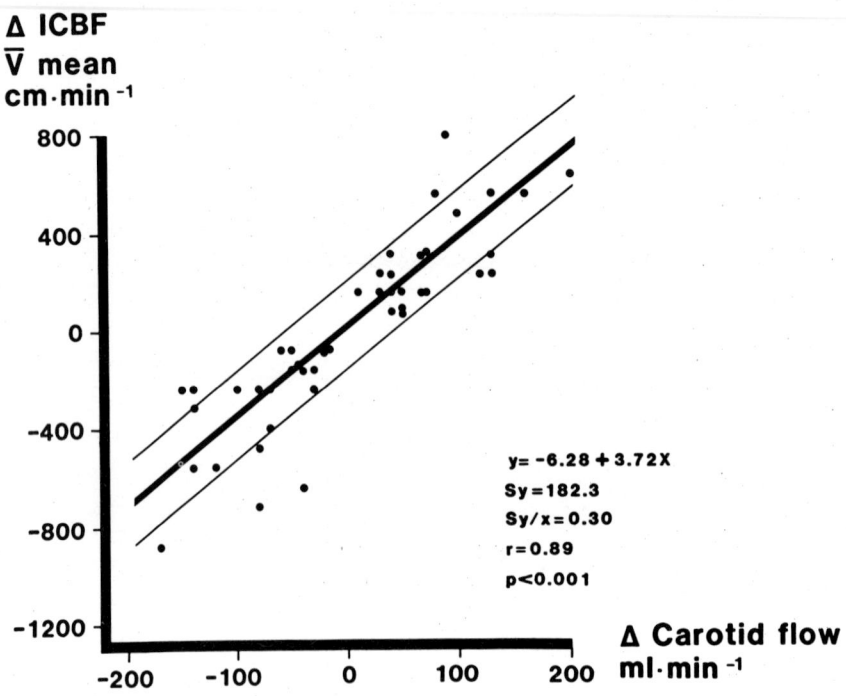

Fig.5. Changes in intracranial blood flow velocity (ICBF) versus changes in carotid blood flow on the same side. Regression line and equation.

Chronic animal model

Newborn lambs were used as study animals. Artificial fontanels were made on both sides of the midline through the skull under general anesthesia. Arterial and venous catheters were also placed. ECG electrodes were placed subcutaneously. The animals were allowed to recover for three days in the ewe´s pens. No other drugs than antibiotics were given.

The lamb was placed standing in a sling at the time of study. A pressure transducer was hooked-up to the arterial catheter and the ECG electrodes to an ECG amplifier. The Doppler crystal was held on the fontanel and the ultrasound beam directed towards a strong arterial flow on the base of the skull. The maximum depth under the fontanel was used and the sampling volume was set at 2 mm longitudinal length. Recordings were always made on both sides and the mean value was used for statistical evaluation. Baseline flow velocities were recorded during the first 45 min before any experiment was started. The lambs rested comfortably in the sling and measurements were often made during sleep.

This experimental set-up has been used for various physiological and pharmacological studies of intracranial hemodynamics in the newborn lamb. The technique allows unlimited number of measurements or continuous measurements of intracranial blood flow velocities. The fontanels have remained open for two to three weeks during which repeated studies have been made. The results of these studies are published elsewhere.

DISCUSSION

The Doppler velocimeter used in this study facilitates the identification of deeply lying intracranial arteries by combining continuous and pulsed modes. The measurements, however, must be made in pulsed mode in order to give range resolution. Post mortem examinations on five lambs showed that the measurements had been made in a major artery on the internal base of the skull. One major artery connects the carotid rete and the circle of Willis (Baldwin, 1963). This artery has a relatively axial direction towards the fontanel on the same side but variations are likely to exist. We have therefore used changes rather than absolute flow velocity values for the statistical analysis. Furthermore, the Doppler velocimeter can only measure changes in arterial inflow to the brain and gives no information on regional blood supply. In spite of the fact that the circle of Willis connects the two sides, there was a close correlation between carotid blood flow on the neck and the intracranial blood flow velocity on the same side.
We conclude that the Doppler velocimeter can be used also in animal studies. It permits frequent or continuous measurements of intracranial blood flow velocities in deeply lying arteries. It should be used for measurements of relative changes only. Furthermore, the technique allows truly non-invasive measurements and is therefore useful in chronic animal experiments where invasive procedures could interfere with the results or the animals not be sacrificed.

REFERENCES

Ahman, P.A.(1983): Relationship between pressure passivity and subependymal/ intraventricular hemorrhage as assessed by pulsed ultrasound. Pediatrics 72, 665-669.
Bada, H.S.(1979): Noninvasive diagnosis of neonatal asphyxia and intraventricular hemorrhage by Doppler ultrasound. J. Pediatr. 95, 775-779.
Batton, D.G.(1983): Regional cerebral blood flow, cerebral blood velocity, and pulsatility index in newborn dogs. Pediatr Res. 17, 908-912.
Baldwin, B.A.(1963): Blood flow in the carotid and vertebral arteries of the sheep and calf. J. Physiol.(London) 167, 448-462.
Gray, P.H.(1983): Continuous wave Doppler ultrasound in evaluation of cerebral blood flow in neonates. Arch. Dis. Child. 58, 677-681.
Hansen, N.B.(1983): Validity of Doppler measurements of anterior cerebral artery blood flow velocity: Correlation with brain blood flow in piglets. Pediatrics 72, 526-531.
Hansen, N.B.(1984): The effects of variations in PaCO2 on brain blood flow and cardiac output in the newborn piglet. Pediatr. Res. 18, 1132-1136.
Lundell, B.P.W.(1984): Neonatal cerebral blood flow velocity I: An in vitro validation of the pulsed Doppler technique. Acta Paediatr. Scand. 73, 810-815.
Martin, C.G.(1982): Abnormal cerebral blood flow patterns in preterm infants with a large patent ductus arteriosus. J. Pediatr. 101, 587-593.
Perlman, J.M.(1983): Suctioning in the preterm infant: Effects on cerebral blood flow velocity, intracranial pressure, and arterial blood pressure. Pediatrics 72, 329-334.
Rolfe, P.(1983): An appraisal of techniques for studying cerebral circulation in the newborn. Acta Paediatr. Scand. Suppl. 311, 5-13.
Rosenberg, A.A.(1985): Comparison of anterior cerebral artery blood flow velocity and cerebral blood flow during hypoxia. Pediatr. Res. 19, 67-70.
Rosenkrantz, T.S.(1984): Cerebral blood flow in the newborn lamb with polycythemia and hyperviscosity. J. Pediatr. 104, 276-280.

RESUME

Le débit sanguin cérébral et sa régulation sont surtout connus grâce aux expérimentations animales employant des techniques invasives. Les méthodes destinées au nouveau-né humain doivent être non-invasives. La vélocimétrie Doppler a récemment été utilisée pour étudier l'hémodynamique intra-cranienne. L'expérience rapportée ici avait pour but de valider un système de vélocimétrie Doppler à impulsions permettant un nombre illimité de mesures non-invasives sur l'animal et sans anesthésie.

L'appareil Doppler incluait un système à impulsions à porte unique et un système continu multifréquence. Après conversion analogue-digitale les résultats ont été obtenus en moyennant les mesures sur 50-100 cycles cardiaques. Le débit était calculé par intégration de la surface située au-dessous de la courbe de vélocité.

La validation _in vitro_ a été réalisée avec le modèle schématisé sur la figure 2. Il existait une excellente corrélation entre le débit réel et le débit mesuré par Doppler (vélocité moyenne x surface de section du vaisseau sanguin artificiel).

La validation _in vivo_ a été faite en expérimentation aiguë sur 6 agneaux nouveau-nés sous anesthésie générale. D'une part les débits carotidiens étaient mesurés par des transducteurs électromagnétiques et modifiés par occlusion partielle à complète des carotides. D'autre part les mesures concomitantes de débit par Doppler étaient relevées sur l'artère intra-cranienne la plus profonde atteinte par la sonde Doppler. Les mesures obtenues par les deux techniques étaient en étroite corrélation (Figure 5).

Enfin, des mesures de débit sanguin cérébral par Doppler pulsé ont été faites en expérimentation de longue durée sur des agneaux nouveau-nés préparés, après 3 jours de récupération post-opératoire, sans anesthésie et souvent en cours de sommeil spontané. Ce modèle a permis des mesures discontinues illimitées ou des mesures continues pendant 2 à 3 semaines (résultats sous presse).

En conclusion, cette méthode permet des mesures des <u>variations relatives</u> de vélocité et non des mesures absolues; cependant la vélocimétrie Doppler relève des modifications du débit artériel arrivant au cerveau mais ne donne aucune information sur les débits régionaux. Toutefois cette technique s'avère utile en expérimentation animale chronique.

Developmental difference in peripheral circulatory response to feeding of newborn and growing preterm infants

A.C. Yao, M.H. Kim, A. Gatmaitan, P. Nuchpuckdee and G. Valencia

Department of Pediatrics, SUNY-Downstate Medical Center, Brooklyn, New York, NY 11203, USA

ABSTRACT

The influence of developmental age on postprandial peripheral circulatory response was investigated in 24 growing preterm (28-36 wks gestation) infants 14-110 days old. They were grouped by postconceptual age (Mean ± S.D.) into (I) 41.1 ± 1.7 wks, n=9, (II) 38.2 ± 0.4 wks, n=9 and (III) 36.3 ± 0.3 wks, n=6. Lower limb blood flow (LBF) was measured by venous occlusion plethysmorgraphic method pre- and postprandially. Blood pressure (BP), pulse rate (PR), skin, rectal and room temperatures were monitored. Peripheral vascular resistance (PVR) was calculated from mean BP and LBF. Milk formula (23 ml/Kg) feeding results in: Group (I) infants, a significant decrease in LBF within 30 min, followed by increases above prefeed level by 60-150 min. PVR varied inversely as the LBF. The findings suggest an initial regional blood flow redistribution. Groups (II) and (III) infants showed no significant changes in LBF and PVR. BP, PR and temperatures did not change significantly in all groups. Thus, infants who attained postconceptual ages of ≥ 39 wks responded to feeding like that reported in normal term neonates and those of 36-38 wks, responded like preterm infants ≤ 2 wks old. The results suggest that postprandial peripheral blood flow changes is developmental age dependent.

Keywords

Developmental age, peripheral circulation, limb blood flow, feeding, postconceptual, preterm infants.

INTRODUCTION

The peripheral blood flow of the newborn infant per unit tissue volume is greater than in adults (Celander, 1966) and it decreased with advancing gestational and postnatal ages (Wu et al, 1980). This difference has been attributed to the larger surface area, more vascularized skin and lower muscle tone, especially in preterm infants.

Feeding induced an initial peripheral vasoconstriction in the term newborn infants, prior to the onset of vasodilation (Yao et al, 1971). It has been suggested that the initial vasoconstriction represents redistribution of peripheral blood flow in favor of increased splanchnic circulatory demand before a more generalized compensatory response could be established. Preterm infants under two weeks old failed to manifest similar peripheral vascular responses with feeding (Raziuddin et al, 1984). A developmental basis for this difference has been postulated.

The purpose of the present study was to examine the influence of developmental age on the postprandial peripheral circulatory changes of preterm infants. To achieve this, we investigated the peripheral blood flow responses to feeding in growing preterm infants of various ages as they approached the postconceptual age of term.

MATERIALS AND METHODS

The subjects were 24 growing preterm infants born at 28-36 weeks gestation with birth weights of 790-1980 gm. At the time of the study, their postnatal age range was 14-110 days, they were clinically well and receiving routine oral feedings in the low risk nursery. They were grouped by postconceptual age into (I) 41.1 ± 1.7 wks (mean ± SD), n=9 (II) 38.2 ± 0.4 wks, n=9, and (III) 36.3 ± 0.3 wks, n=6. The body weights of the babies of the three groups were comparable (Table I).

Parental consent was obtained and the protocol was approved by the local ethics committee.

Lower limb blood flow (LBF) was measured by venous occlusion plethysmographic method using an air-filled latex double-walled plethysmographic cuff, fitted snugly to the midportion of the calf, and the occlusion applied via a blood pressure cuff around the lower thigh. Details of the technique was described previously (Wallgren 1967, Raziuddin et al 1984). The LBF was recorded 30 min before and half-hourly for 2½ hours after feeding. The mean of three consecutive technically good tracings was taken as representative of the LBF which was expressed in ml/min/100 ml tissue.

Blood pressure was measured by the Doppler ultrasound technique (Roche Arteriosonde Model 1010) and pulse rate was obtained from the blood flow tracing. Mean BP was calculated from the mean of the systolic pressure plus twice the diastolic pressure. Peripheral vascular resistance (PVR) was calculated from the mean BP and LBF and expressed in peripheral resistance units (PRU).

The infants were studied in an incubator with servo-control to maintain abdominal skin temperature at $36.5^\circ C$. Rectal and contralateral leg skin temperatures (T) were monitored. These T remained relatively constant throughout the study period. Room T was kept at $26^\circ-27^\circ C$ and it stayed constant during each study.

Feeding consisted of standard commercial milk formula. The amounts were determined by the primary physicians.

Analysis of variance for repeated measure and student's t test were used for data analysis. The p value of $<.05$ was accepted as level of significance. Values were expressed in Mean ± SD.

RESULTS

The clinical data are summarized in Table 1.

TABLE 1. CLINICAL DATA

GROUPS	n	Gest. Age (wks)	Birth Wt. (g)	P.C. Age (wks)	Body Wt. (g)	Amounts Fed (ml/kg)
I	9	31.3 ± 2.2	1226.1 ±436	41.1 ± 1.7	2128.9 ±347	24.0 ± 5.4
II	9	35.3 ± 0.9	1728.3 ±292	38.2 ± 0.4	2117.0 ±190	22.5 ± 5.2
III	6	31.5 ± 2.4	1450.0 ±324	36.3 ± 0.3	1926.7 ±289	23.5 ± 5.4

P.C. postconceptual, values are mean ± SD, gest. gestation, wt. weight.

There were no significant differences in the amount of feeding taken by infants amongst the groups (see Table 1). The mean body weight was not different amongst the 3 groups in spite of the difference in PC age. However, there was wider scatter of weights within groups I and III.

Pulse rate, mean BP values are shown in Fig. 1. Group 1 infants, who were older, had slightly lower PR and higher mean BP than groups II and III. The difference however, was not statistically significant. No significant changes in PR and mean BP occurred postprandially in all groups.

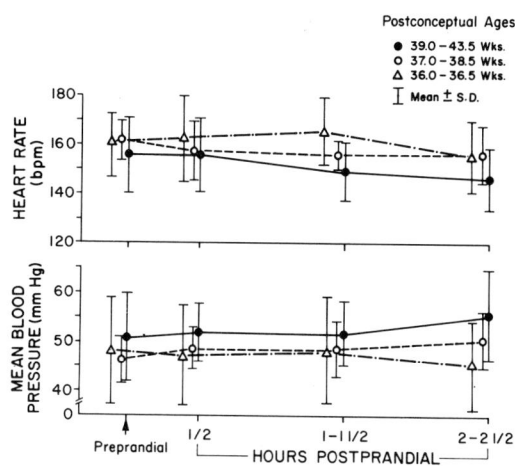

Fig. 1. Effect of feeding on the mean blood pressure and heart rate of 24 growing preterm infants of different postconceptual ages. No significant changes occurred in all three groups postprandially.

The LBF and PVR changes are shown in Figs. 2 and 3. The prefeed control LBF value of group I was higher than in group II but not in group III. The control PVR was not different between the groups. The mean LBF of group I infants decreased significantly by 25% from prefeed value (14.3 ± 2.9 ml/min/100 ml) at ½ hour postprandially. This was followed by an increase (35%) at the 60-90 min measurement which persisted through 120-150 min (Fig. 2). Only 3 infants in group II and 1 in Group III showed similar patterns of postprandial LBF changes, all others in these two groups showed insignificant increase in LBF after feeding. Thus, as groups, both II and III showed no significant LBF changes after feeding. The postprandial LBF changes were significantly different between groups I and II (P<.015) and I and III (P<.05) at 30 min but not subsequently. In group I the PVR increased by 32% from the prefeed value (3.66 ± 0.9 PRU) 30 mins after feeding which paralleled the LBF decrease (see Fig. 3). This was followed by PVR decreases (14-20%) at 60 min and 120 min as the LBF increased (Fig. 2). Groups II and III infants showed no significant postprandial changes in PVR. The PVR changes at 30 min was different between groups I and II (P=.05) and groups I and III (p <.05).

There were no significant changes in skin and rectal temperatures in infants of all groups.

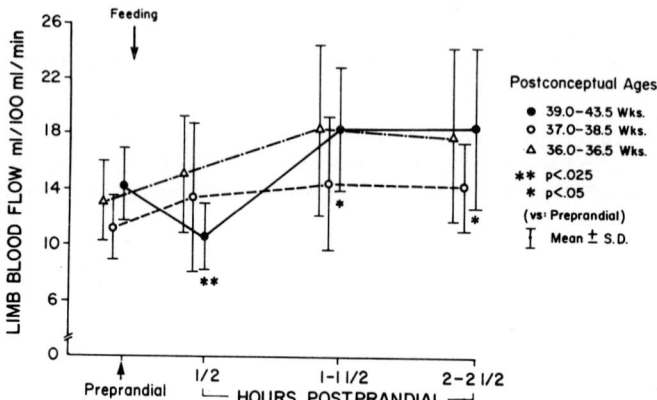

Fig. 2. Effect of feeding on limb blood flow of 24 growing preterm infants of different postconceptual (PC) ages. Significant postprandial changes occurred in infants ≥39 wks PC age, i.e. a decrease at ½ hour and increases at 1-1½ hour and 2-2½ hour measurements. No significant changes occurred in infants ≤38.5 wks. PC ages.

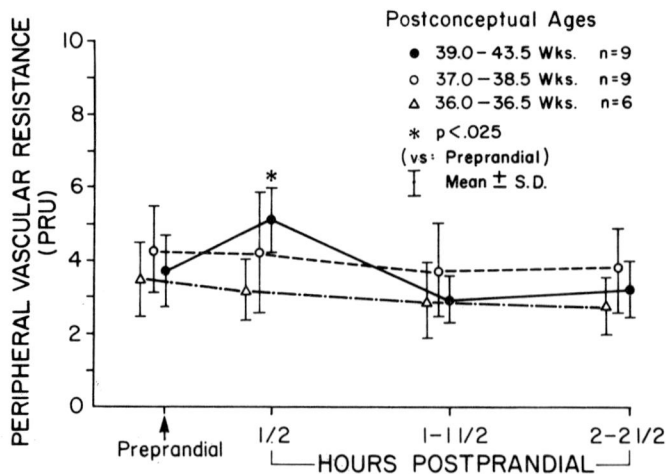

Fig. 3. Effect of feeding on the peripheral vascular resistance (PVR) of 24 growing preterm infants of different postconceptual (PC) ages. Infants ≥39 wks PC age showed a significant increase of PVR at ½ hr following feeding which decreased to below control values after 1-1½ hours. Infants ≤38.5 wks PC ages showed no significant changes.

DISCUSSION

The prefeed LBF was higher than our previous values of preterm infants under 2 weeks old. This appeared contrary to the observed decreasing LBF with advancing postnatal age (Wu et al 1980). The reasons for this discrepancy are probably related to the wide range in postnatal and gestational ages, the small for date weight status, especially in group I infants who had the highest value and should not affect our results because we measured longitudinal changes in blood flow and compared the blood flow changes between groups.

Like normal term neonates (Yao et al 1971), the postprandial peripheral circulatory response in group I infants, who had attained term PC ages was an initial increase in peripheral vascular resistance with decreased LBF, followed by vasodilation and increased LBF 1-2½ hrs after feeding. This occurred in the infants in spite of their lower than full term body weight. The findings were consistent with that reported in the week-old term, small for gestational age, low birth weight infants (Raziuddin et al 1984). Conversely, the lack of postprandial LBF changes in groups II and III infants (PC ages 36-38 wks) were comparable to results in 1-2 wk old preterm infants (Raziuddin et al 1984) despite their older postnatal age. These results suggest that postnatal age per se was not as significant a factor as PC age or maturity in influencing the newborn or preterm infants' peripheral vascular responses to feeding.

The mechanisms involved in these vascular changes were not within the scope of this study. However, we speculate that factors controlling the peripheral vasomotor tone follow an age related maturational process. Although extrapolation from animal studies is limited by species difference, it is of interest that Buckley et al (1981a, 1981b) had demonstrated the absence of tonic sympathetic vasoconstrictor tone in the femoral vasculature of a day old piglet. We have found postprandial femoral vasoconstriction in piglets 2-4 wks old but not in those <2 days old. Peripheral blood flow was shown to be considerably affected by the enhanced sympathoadrenal activity at birth (Faxelius et al, 1984), and the magnitude of catecholamine release in infants with birth asphyxia was found to be gestational age related (Lagercrantz 1971). Catecholamines were not measured in the present study. Their influence on the peripheral circulation postprandially, and those of the other gastrointestinal vasoactive hormones remained to be investigated in term and preterm neonates.

In spite of an active peripheral vasomotor controlling system, newborn term infants have shown a decreased capacity to maintain circulatory homeostasis under hypo- and hypervolemia (Wallgren et al, 1964, 1967). It thus appeared reasonable to expect a less well-developed circulatory controlling system of preterm infants. Based on the results of this study it is tempting to speculate that the preterm infant may be at a disadvantage when their gastrointestinal blood flow demand is challenged. Their inability to call on the peripheral vascular compensatory mechanism may predispose them to intestinal pathology like necrotizing enterocolitis.

Intestinal oxidative demands could be met by local mechanisms like increased oxygen extraction rather than increased blood flow as found in the newborn lambs (Edelstone et al 1981). Newborn piglets however responded by both increased blood flow and O_2 extraction (Nowicki et al, 1983). Similar mechanism may operate in the newborn and preterm infants.

In summary, the results of this study indicate that feeding induced no significant changes in LBF of infants 36-38 wks in postconceptual age like younger preterm infants. In contrast, preterm infants who attained postconceptual age of 39 weeks or greater responded to feeding like normal term infants, by an initial increase in peripheral vascular resistance with decreased LBF followed by vasodilation and increased LBF. The peripheral blood flow response to feeding in preterm infants is thus developmental age dependent.

REFERENCES

Buckley, N.M., Brazeau, P., Frasier, I.D., Gootman, P.M. (1981a): Femoral circulatory responses to lumbar nerve stimulation in developing swine. Am. J. Physiol. 240:H505-H510.

Buckley, N.M., Brazeau, P., Frasier, I.D., Gootman, P.M. (1981b): Maturation of circulatory responses to adrenergic stimuli. Fed. Proc. 42:1643-1647.

Celander, O. (1980): Studies of the peripheral circulation. In The Heart and Circulation In the Newborn Infant, Cassels, D.E., ed., pp 98-110, New York Grune & Stratton.

Edelstone, D.I., Holzman, I.R. (1981): Gastrointestinal tract O_2 uptake and regional blood flows during digestion in conscious newborn lambs. Am. J. Physiol. 241:G289-G293.

Faxelius, G., Lagercrantz, H., Yao, A.C. (1984): Sympathoadrenal activity and peripheral blood flow after birth: comparison in infants delivered vaginally and by cesarean section. 105:144-148.

Lagercrantz, H., Bistoletti, P. (1977): Catecholamine release in the newborn infants at birth. Pediatr. Res. 11:889-893.

Nowicki, P., Stonestreet, B.S., Hansen, N., Yao, A.C., Oh, W. (1983): Gastrointestinal blood flow and oxygen consumption in awake newborn piglets: effect of feeding. Am. J. Physiol. 245:G697-G702.

Raziuddin, K., Kim, M.H., Yao, A.C. (1984): Peripheral circulatory response to feeding in newborn low-birth-weight infants. J. Pediatr. Gastroenterol. Nutrition 3:89-94.

Wallgren G., Lind, J. (1967): Quantitative studies of the human neonatal circulation. IV Observations on the newborn infants' peripheral circulation and plasma expansion during moderate hypovolemia. Acta. Paediatr Scand Suppl 179:55-68.

Wallgren, G., Barr, M., Rudhe, U. (1964): Hemodynamic studies of induced acute hypo- and hypervolemia in the newborn infant. Acta. Paediatr Scand 53:1-12.

Wu, P.Y.K., Wong, W.H., Guerra, G., Miranda, R., Godoy, R.R., Preston, B., Schoentgen, S. and Levan, N.E. (1980): Peripheral blood flow in the neonate. 1. Changes in total, skin, and muscle blood flow with gestational and postnatal age. Pediatr. Res. 14:1374-1378.

Yao, A.C., Wallgren, C.G., Sinha, S.N., Lind, J. (1971): Peripheral circulatory responses to feeding in the newborn infant. Pediatr. 47:378-382

Address queries to:

> Dr. Alice C. Yao
> Department of Pediatrics
> Downstate Medical Center, Box 49
> 450 Clarkson Avenue
> Brooklyn, New York 11203   U.S.A.

RESUME

Le débit sanguin périphérique rapporté à l'unité de volume de tissu est plus élevé chez le nouveau-né que chez l'adulte; il diminue en raison inverse de l'âge gestationnel et de l'âge post-natal. Chez le nouveau-né à terme, les repas sont suivis d'abord d'une vasoconstriction périphérique puis d'une vasodilatation. Cette vasocontriction initiale pourrait correspondre à une redistribution du débit sanguin périphérique au profit de la circulation splanchnique alors sollicitée. Cette réaction n'a pas été observée chez le prématuré. L'étude rapportée ici a donc été conçue pour analyser l'influence de l'âge maturatif sur la réponse circulatoire périphérique en période post-prandiale.

La série comprend 24 prématurés nés entre 28 et 36 semaines de gestation, d'un poids de naissance de 790-1980 gm, et âgés de 14-110 jours de vie. Le groupe I (n=9) a un âge conceptionnel de $41,1 \pm 1,7$ semaines, le groupe II (n=9) $38,2 \pm 0,4$ semaines, et le groupe III (n=6) $36,3 \pm 0,3$ semaines. La mesure du débit sanguin dans un membre inférieur est réalisée par pléthysmographie à partir d'un brassard de mesure fixé à mi-mollet, tandis que l'occlusion veineuse est obtenue par un brassard de prise de pression artérielle appliqué à la cuisse. La mesure de débit est faite 30 minutes avant un repas et toutes les 30 minutes pendant les 2 heures 1/2 suivant le repas. Le résultat est exprimé en ml/min/100ml de tissu. La pression artérielle, la fréquence cardiaque, et les températures cutanées, rectales, et ambiantes, sont enregistrées. Le repas administré est celui prescrit par le pédiatre responsable de l'enfant. La résistance vasculaire périphérique (RVP) est calculée à partir de la pression artérielle moyenne et du débit sanguin dans le membre inférieur (DSMI).

Après un repas d'un volume moyen de 23ml/Kg, les résultats ont été les suivants: 1) Dans le groupe I, le DSMI diminue de façon significative dans les 30 premières minutes suivant le repas, puis s'élève de nouveau et dépasse le niveau de base pré-prandial vers la 60-150e minute. La RVP varie en raison inverse du DSMI. Ces observations suggèrent l'existence d'une redistribution initiale du débit sanguin régional. 2) Dans les groupes II et III, il n'a été observé aucune variation significative du DSMI ni de la RVP. Dans aucun des 3 groupes, il n'y a eu de variation significative de la pression artérielle, ni de la fréquence cardiaque, ni des températures.

Par conséquent, les enfants ayant atteint l'âge conceptionnel d'au moins 39 semaines réagissent à un repas de la même façon que les nouveau-nés à terme normaux; les enfants d'un âge conceptionnel de 36-38 semaines réagissent comme les prématurés âgés de 2 semaines décrits par Razzuidin et al. (1984). Ces résultats laissent penser que les modifications post-prandiales du débit sanguin périphérique sont fonction de l'âge conceptionnel.

DISCUSSION. Pr.P.Karlberg moderator.

Dr.W.Oh: Do you think that the younger subjects are more efficient in terms of the mesenteric response than the older ones or is it the other way around?

Dr.A.Yao: It is rather the other way around. Of course, we only measured peripheral blood flow, not mesenteric blood flow, therefore the finding is subject to different interpretation. We interpreted the changes in peripheral flow as an indirect reflection of the increased splanchnic oxidative demand. The fact that the term infants decreased their peripheral blood flow in the early postprandial period suggested to us that perhaps they redistribute their peripheral flow in favor of feeding induced increased splanchnic flow. The premature infants, however, did not do that; perhaps they were unable to do so; maybe their peripheral vasomotor tone was not "mature".

Dr.J.Metcoff: One of the first slides showed post-conceptual weights in the range of 2100g for 41 weeks. I wonder whether that represented significant malnutrition in these babies? And whether that degree of malnutrition also occurred in the samll-for-gestational-age babies (SGA) you showed later. The similarities between the two suggest that the low birthweight was not attributable to gestational age but to the nutritional state. What were the actual birthweights and gestational ages of that first group of babies?

Dr.A.Yao: That is a very well-taken point. What lead us to think that the response is age-related is that perfectly normal full-term infants behave this same way. So it is hard to think that weight or nutritional state would be the main determining factor.

Dr.B.Lundell: Did you look at repeated feeding? Are there differences between the breast-fed, bottle-fed as compared to the tube-fed babies?

Dr.A.Yao: In the very first study we did with Dr.Göran Wallgren in term infants (Pediatrics 1971,$\underline{47}$:378), all were breast-fed full-term babies. The response was similar to that of bottle-fed infants. In that group we had tried repeated feeding in a few infants and they responded the same way each time.

Dr.B.Friis-Hansen: Have you done any research on whether this response is being mediated by catecholamines?

Dr.A.Yao: We are planning to do catecholamines and the vasoactive peptides.

Dr.Ab.Rudolph.: These results are interesting in regard to the redistribution of blood flow. It has been shown in newborn lambs that gastrointestinal blood does not increase much in response to feeding. The increase in gastrointestinal oxygen consumption after feeding is largely associated with an increase in oxygen extraction rather than an increase of blood flow (Edelstone & Holzman, Amer J Physiol 1981, $\underline{241}$: G289).

Dr.A.Yao: Together with the group in Providence (Amer J Physiol 1983, $\underline{245}$: G697) we did a similar work in newborn piglets. There we found both flow and oxygen consumption increased with feeding. Maybe there is a species difference.

Gastrointestinal hormones in newborn infants: release mechanisms and possible circulatory effects

G. Marchini, H. Lagercrantz, J. Winberg and K. Uvnäs-Moberg

Department of Pediatrics, Karolinska Hospital, and Department of Pharmacology, Karolinska Institute, Stockholm, Sweden

ABSTRACT.

Some gastro-intestinal hormones were assayed in blood samples from infants during non-nutritive suckling and during sensory stimulation of the cheek (rooting reflex). The aim was to investigate the role of vagal activation for gastro-intestinal hormone release.

Blood samples were collected from the umbilical artery or vein in infants with indwelling catheters due to transient respiratory problems and polycytemia respectively. Insulin was found to rise significantly in nine out of seventeen suckling infants, and gastrin in two of fourteen. In some of the infants with lack of gastrin release, high somatostatin levels were found. Elicitation of the rooting reflex was found to trigger a significant release of insulin and oxytocin.

We have found that vagal activation by non-nutritive suckling or sensory stimulation is important for the release of gastro-intestinal hormones, suggesting that early breast-feeding should be promoted. These hormones stimulate the growth of the gastric and intestinal mucosa. Some of the gastro-intestinal hormones like vasoactive intestinal polypeptide (released by oxytocin and gastrin) have also substantial circulatory effects, shunting blood towards the gastro-intestinal tract.

NOTE
Dr. Marchini et al. apologize for not being able to provide a full length paper within schedule.

RESUME.

Des dosages de certaines hormones gastro-intestinales ont été effectués sur des prélèvements sanguins obtenus chez des nouveau-nés pendant la succion non-nutritive et au cours de la stimulation sensorielle de la joue (recherche du réflexe des points cardinaux).. Cette étude avait pour but de rechercher le rôle de l'activation vagale dans la libération des hormones gastro-intestinales.

Les prélèvements sanguins ont été recueillis à partir de l'artère ou de la veine ombilicale, par des cathéters à demeure posés en raison soit d'une détresse respiratoire transitoire, soit d'une polycythémie. Il a été observé une montée **significative** du taux d'insuline chez 9 des nourrissons pendant la succion, et une élévation de la gastrine chez deux nourrissons sur 14. Chez certains nouveau-nés ne présentant pas de libération de gastrine, on a relevé des taux importants de somatostatine. La recherche des points cardinaux a déclenché une libération significative d'insuline et d'ocytocine.

Selon cette étude, l'activation vagale consécutive à la succion non-nutritive ou à la stimulation sensorielle est importante pour la libération des hormones gastro-intestinales, résultat qui fait penser que l'allaitement précoce devrait être encouragé. Ces hormones stimulent la croissance de la muqueuse gastrique et intestinale. Certaines hormones gastro-intestinales telles que le VIP ("vasoactive intestinal polypeptide"), libéré par l'ocytocine et la gastrine, ont aussi des effets circulatoires non-négligeables, en favorisant le débit sanguin en direction du tractus digestif.

****

DISCUSSION. Dr.W.Oh moderator

<u>Dr.J.Warshaw</u>: You have about 20 years of work ahead of you looking at all the variables that affect these hormones. Clinical situations such as the short gut syndrome raise important questions. There are also factors such as fatty acids which have been suggested to contribute to the hypertrophic response as well as epidermal growth factor (EGF) and perhaps other factors in milk. Have you looked into any of these to see whether milk itself or components of milk stimulate a response?

<u>Dr.G.Marchini</u>: No, we did not. Our study only involved <u>non-nutritive</u> suckling.

<u>Dr.W.Oh</u>: What are the hormonal variations, particularly insulin for instance, within the 6-minute period, without any suckling, just picking up the baby?

<u>Dr.G.Marchini</u>: We are looking at that right now in control groups.

<u>Dr.B.Friis-Hansen</u>: Would you recommand that a premature baby on continuous tube feeding should be given a sucking possibility?

<u>Dr.G.Marchini</u>: Why not? It has already been done by Bernbaum et al. (Pediatrics 1983, <u>71</u>:41); their study showed that the intestinal transit time was decreased when premature babies suckled during tube feeding. A more recent study by Paludetto et al. also demonstrated an increased transcutaneous oxygen tension during non-nutritive suckling (Pediatrics 1984, <u>74</u>:539).

<u>Dr.W.Oh</u>: In a study from our group, we have demonstrated an accelerated gastric emptying when the babies were allowed to suck.

<u>Dr.Ab.Rudolph</u>: How long does the response last? If one repeats suckling, do second and third responses occur? Does the response to repetitive suckling wear off?

<u>Dr.G.Marchini</u>: We just looked into what happened within 5 minutes and

there was just one peak. The problem lies with the number of samples that you can take from a baby, which is limited. With electrical stimulation of a nerve, a similar pattern is observed: a certain time has to pass before repeating the experiment to get the same response.

<u>Dr. J. Metcoff</u>: How does this particular phenomenon help the maturation process?

<u>Dr. G. Marchini</u>: That was mainly taught by the gastrin. In rats, it stimulates cellular proliferation in the gastro-intestinal tract. However, this has been demonstrated in rats, not in humans.

Onset of breathing, respiratory adaptation, surfactant
Installation de la respiration, adaptation respiratoire, surfactant

Respiratory control during onset of breathing

P. Karlberg and G. Wennergren

Göteborg University, Department of Pediatrics I, East Hospital, S-416 85 Göteborg, Sweden

ABSTRACT

At birth several drastic functional changes occur, of which the onset of air breathing is the key issue. There, the change in blood oxygen level from a low fetal to a high extrauterine level represents the most essential adaptation. The start of respiration is elicited by several cooperating stimuli, biochemical via CO_2 accumulation and metabolic acidosis, and sensory via tactile and cold receptors as well as auditory and visual stimuli. Enhanced alertness via increased catecholamine levels probably acts as a facilitating factor. An important role for the establishment of a regular breathing seems to be played by an excitatory drive from the central and peripheral chemoreceptors. In contrast to the excitatory respiratory drive provided by the transient CO_2 rise at birth, hypoxia as a net effect has a depressory influence on respiration in the just newborn infant. Also, the central nervous structures effectuating the respiratory control are discussed.

KEY WORDS

Onset of breathing, respiratory control, apnea, periodic breathing, hypoxia, hypercapnia, central and peripheral chemoreceptors, sensory stimuli, cathecholamines.

INTRODUCTION

The transition from intrauterine to extrauterine existence implies drastic functional changes. A successful and smooth transition to demands ready and alert breathing control mechanisms. The most dramatic event is the onset of air breathing followed by continuous, regular breathing, thereby altering placental gas exchange to pulmonary. The lungs are ready and prepared for an effective gas exchange, however, still filled with lung fluid. On the other hand the control mechanisms for this breathing are different than those for the respiratory movements during the fetal life. The fetal respiration is constituted by rapid, shallow respiratory movements which (in sheep) are associated with the periods of active sleep (Dawes et al, 1972) and not primarily with biochemical stimuli.

Before birth the fetus lies surrounded by amniotic water, swimming around, warm and weight less. It listens to its mother's pulse but sensory inputs from the external world in terms of sound and light are dampened and low-key. All needs of the fetus are taken care of via the umbilical cord. Labour and delivery abruptly terminates this state as the fetus is

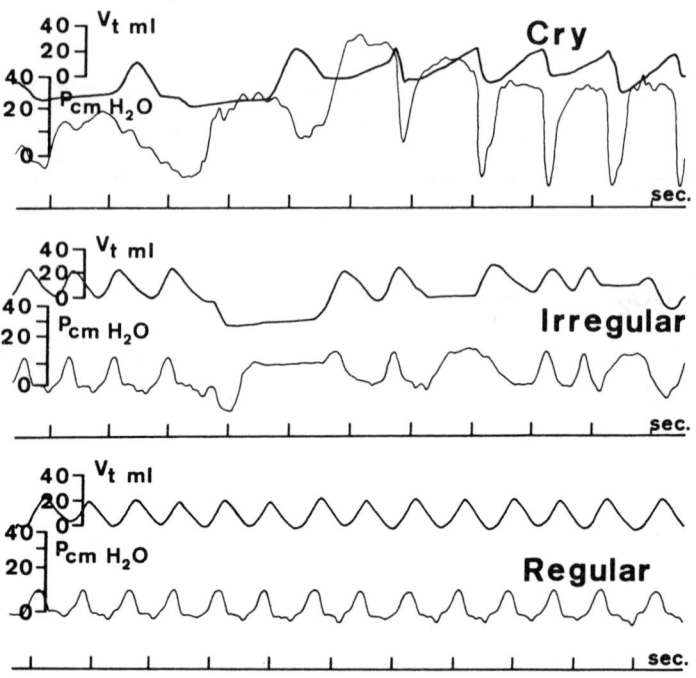

Fig. 1. The three respiratory patterns found in the first 15 minutes after birth. The intraesophageal pressure changes may be seen in the lower part of the tracing (from Engström et al, 1966 in. Onset of respiration. Association for the aid of crippled children, New York).

pushed and squeezed through the birth canal. A state of harmony is replaced by a state of stress (cf Lagercrantz and Bistoletti, 1977) but also of alertness.

Within the first 10-20 seconds after birth the newborn normally takes his first, large breath which then is followed by, at the start usually irregular breathing with interposed pauses, but then soon regular breathing, see Fig. 1, (Karlberg et al, 1962; Engström et al, 1966). Several most important events shall take place in a rapid sequence. With the first breath the replacement of the lung fluid with air starts, at vaginal delivery supported by the thoracic squeeze and following recoil (Karlberg 1960, 1985). Already during the first minute a gas exchange takes place with O_2 up-take and CO_2 output (Karlberg and Celander, 1965 a). This means also that the hitherto low pulmonary blood perfusion is rapidly increasing. In a normal situation, a well functioning pulmonary respiration at a balanced steady state is established within 10-20 minutes (Tunell et al, 1976).

The events are important to analyze since the arrival of the newborn to extrauterine life is not always uncomplicated. When the onset of breathing does not occur in a normal way, there is risk of ultimate damage to the central nervous system. However, the establishment of air breathing is initiated by several cooperating stimuli of both sensory and biochemical nature. In this paper the discussion will be focused on the respiratory control during onset of breathing.

ONSET OF BREATHING
CHANGES IN RESP. AND NON-RESP. FACTORS

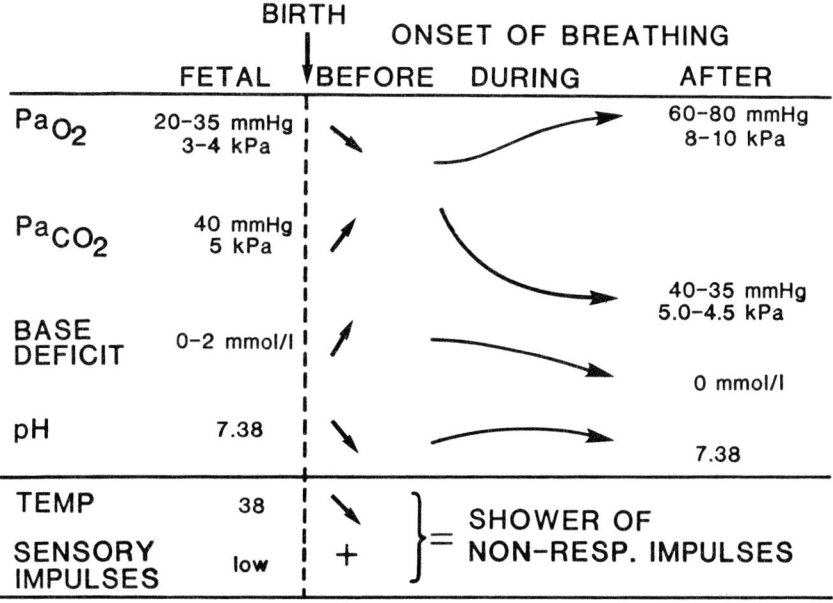

Fig. 2. Graphically illustrated changes in respiratory and non-respiratory factors at onset of breathing.

STARTING POINT OF THE ONSET OF BREATHING

The fetal situation is outlined in Fig. 2. Fetal PCO_2 is about 5 kPa and PO_2 is approximately 3-4.5 with a base deficit of 0-2 and pH 7.38.

The stress exerted on the fetus by the labour and compression of the cord may have accomplished a more or less disturbed gas exchange with accumulation of carbon dioxide as well as impairment of the oxygenation with developing metabolic acidosis.

BIOCHEMICAL EVENTS AND STIMULI

With a situation where breathing has not yet started, while the placental circulation is ceasing, there will be a climb in the newborn's PCO_2, a drop in PO_2 and a building up of respiratory as well as metabolic acidosis. When the first breath is elicited, there will be a blow off of CO_2, lowering the arterial PCO_2 level. However, until regular breathing is established, PCO_2 will start climbing again and PO_2 as well as pH will fall. The rising PCO_2 will provide an excitatory influence on respiratory neurons via stimulation of the central, ventral medullary chemoreceptors. The combined hypercapnia, hypoxia and acidosis will act exciting via stimulation of the peripheral chemoreceptors. These, however, probably not yet has been reset to operate in the sensitivity range they will have later, with a new set-point in the high PO_2-range appropriate for the air breathing situation (Blanco et al, 1984; Grögaard, 1982, 1983). A situation with sufficiently strong biochemical stimulation will

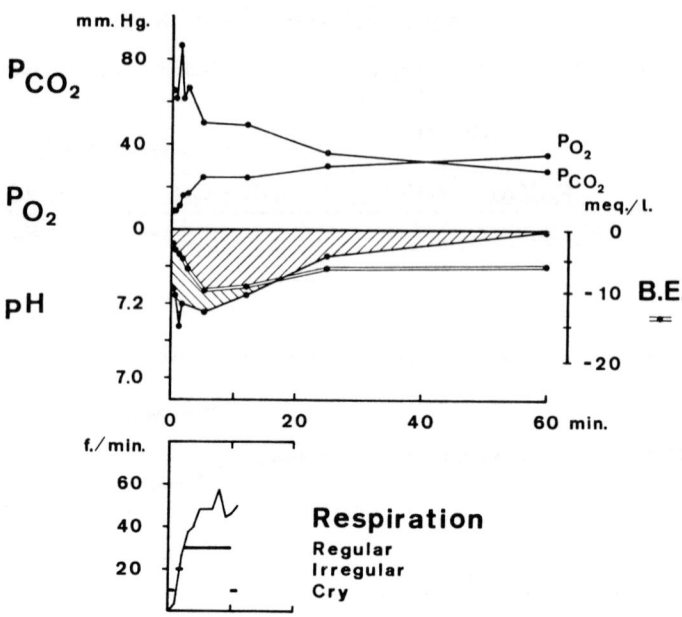

Fig. 3. Iliac-arterry blood gas tension, acid-base balance, and respiratory recordings in a newborn infant from birth up to 60 min (from Engström, et al, 1966, in: Onset of respiration. Association for the aid of crippled children, New York).

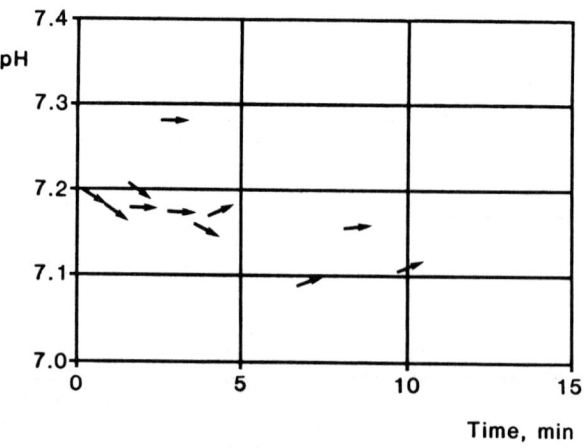

Fig. 4. Arterial pH at start of regular respiration with medium tidal volume, based on the results in the study of Engström et al (1966).

however soon be reached providing a substantial part of the respiratory drive that establishes a normal an regular respiration. A series of repeated blood-gas and acid-base measurements immediately after birth by Engström et al (1966) illustrates this. An example is graphically illustrated in Fig. 3. In a series of 25 newborns it was found that there was a fall in pH down to about 7.18 before regular breathing started, see Fig. 4. With improved oxygenation the PCO_2 soon will be controlled down to around 5 kPa and the metabolic acidosis will slowly be metabolized.

A similar pattern was also found by Magno et al (1975, 1976 a, 1976 b) and Kjellmer et al (1974) in 65 infants delivered with Cesarean section where blood-gas and acid-base measurements were obtained immediately at birth (umbilical vein) and at 3, 10, 30, 60 and 120 minutes after delivery. Almost all 65 children had a fall in pH down to 7.20-7.15 before the PO_2 level started to rise, see Fig. 5 a, b, c. The overall inhibitory action of a low oxygen level on respiratory control in the neonate (Cross and Oppé, 1952; Rigatto and Brady, 1972 a) makes it reasonable to postulate that at a PO_2 level of 3-4 kPa, regular breathing is established when that action is balanced off by a combination of overriding excitatory stimuli of both biochemical and sensory nature.

SENSORY STIMULI

A shower of sensory inputs provide stimuli for the first breath, visual, tactile and thermal. The importance of stimulation of cold receptors is illustrated by the following episode noticed by one of us (Karlberg, 1958) a long time ago. Submerging a healthy, breathing newborn baby 1-2 minutes after birth into warm water (head above the water), stopped his breathing. When the baby was taken up from the warm water he started breathing again, when he was immersed, breathing stopped. After the third time the head midwife stopped the manoeuvre. Gluckman et al (1983) has recently in elegant experiments in sheep analyzed this mechanism in detail and convincingly showed how cooling of the lamb fetus elicits breathing. Massage and perhaps a gentle spanking of the baby will stimulate onset of breathing in a similar way.

CATHECHOLAMINE STIMULI

The cathecholamine surge elicited in the baby during the labour (Lagercrantz and Bistoletti, 1977) produces an increased alertness which was clearly experienced in a study in newborn infants some days old, where the primary aim was to study the influence on metabolism by noradrenaline (Karlberg et al, 1965 b). Noradrenaline given i.v. made the babies so alert that a steady state level was difficult to obtain. Such an alertness probably provides a background excitation in the brain stem which facilitates breathing activity. Furthermore, the turn off of lung liquid production is mediated via stimulation of beta-receptors (Walters and Olver, 1978). Hence an increased cathecholamine level probably contributes to reversing lung liquid production into resorption, thereby promoting respiratory adaptation. Existence of established labour activity with rupture of membranes before birth with Cesarean delivery, per se decreases the risk for respiratory adaptation disturbances of type transient tachypnea of the newborn (e.g. Wennergren, M. et al, 1985).

NEURAL STRUCTURES EFFECTUATING THE RESPIRATORY CONTROL

How are then the neural structures organized that effectuate the respiratory control (von Euler, 1985). The basic breathing pattern is constituted of rhythmic variations in inspiratory activity. The important groups of inspiratory neurons are located in two parts of the medulla oblongata. Dorsally in the nucleus tractus solitarius, the so-called dorsal respiratory group (DRG) is found. The so-called ventral respiratory group (VRG) is located ventro-laterally, in nucleus paraambigualis. These premotor neurons project down the spinal cord after having crossed the midline and drive the phrenic neurons to the diaphragm and the intercostal

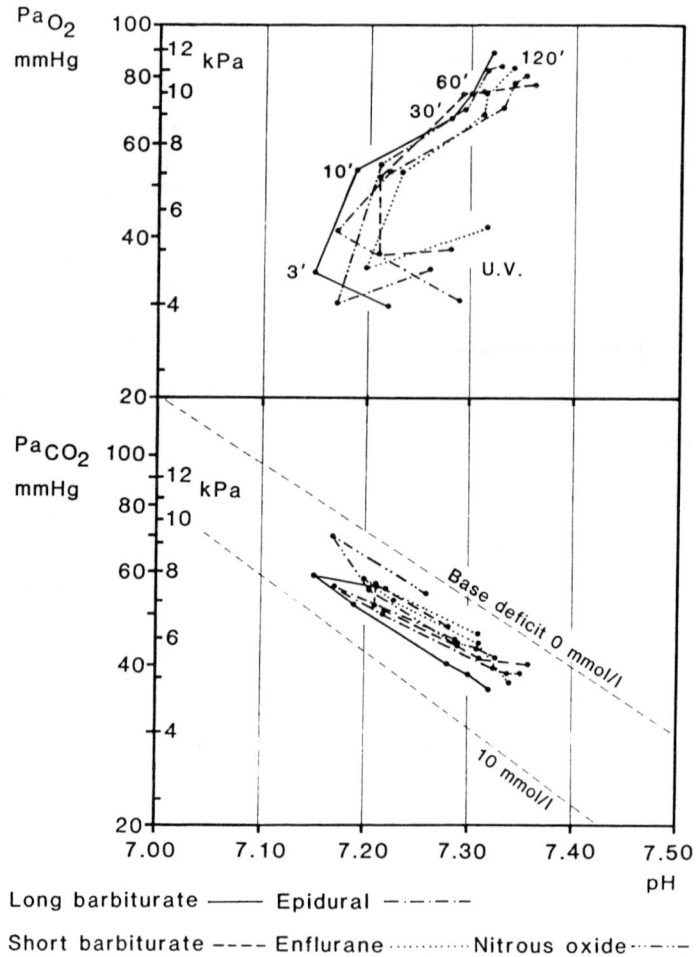

Fig. 5 a. Blood gas changes during and after onset of breathing in newborn infants after Cesarean section after anesthesia with epidural, enflurane, nitrous oxide, long- and short-acting barbiturate, respectively. Blood samples were taken from the umbilical vein immediately at delivery and from the abdominal aorta at 3, 10, 30, 60 and 120 minutes after delivery. The lower part of the graph shows the relationship between $PaCO_2$, base deficit and pH, and the upper part of the graph the relationship between PaO_2 and pH. The relationship between PaO_2 and $PaCO_2$ can be followed via the corresponding pH value. The analysis is performed on original values from Magno et al (1975, 1976 a, b) and Kjellmer et al (1974). In this Fig. the mean values of the five groups are presented.

muscle neurons. Adjacent to the nucleus paraambigualis, in the nucleus ambiguus, the neurons controlling the adductor muscles of the larynx are found. They are most important in the control of air flow during expiration where increased laryngeal adductor muscle activity usually during the first breaths and in the infant with respiratory distress can be heard as grunting.

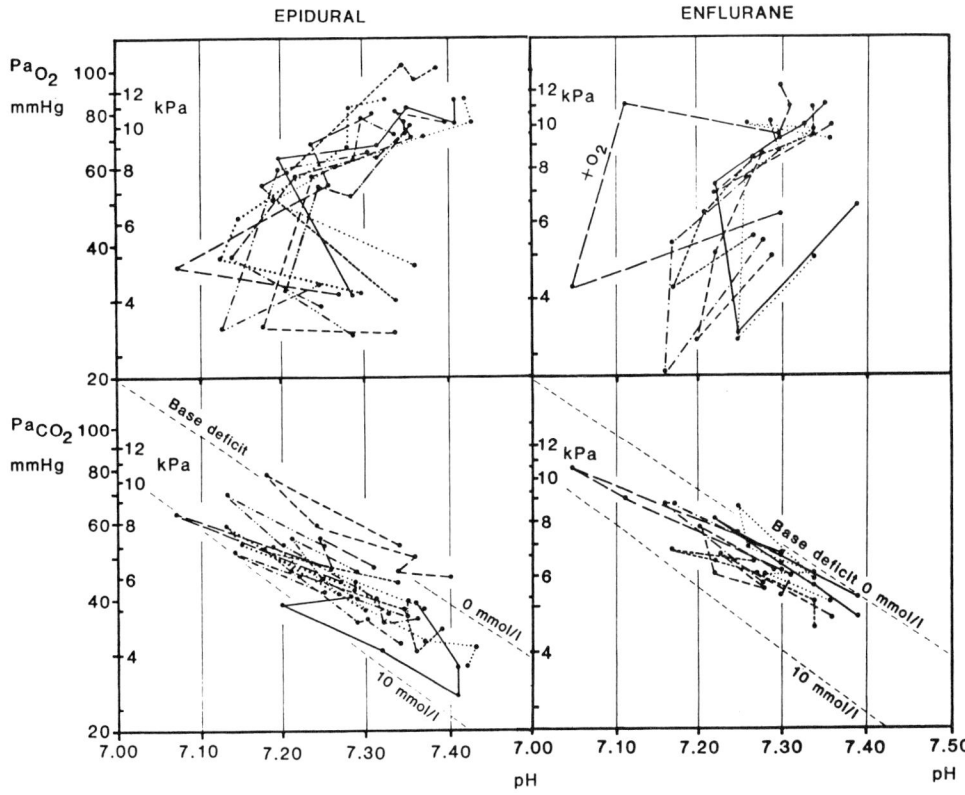

Fig. 5 b and c. Epidural and Enflurane groups. Individual values. See Fig. 5 a.

The expiration related neurons are found in nucleus retroambigualis in the caudal VRG and in the rostral part of VRG.

It is necessary for the inspiratory neurons to receive a tonic driving excitatory influence to be able to maintain a rhythmic breathing pattern. During the awake state such an excitatory input is created by e.g. vision, hearing, thermal and tactile receptors. On the other hand during quiet sleep, the excitatory input is provided by the peripheral, arterial chemoreceptors and by the central chemoreceptors on the ventral surface of the medulla oblongata. The integration of this driving central inspiratory activity takes place in, and just rostro-lateral of, the nucleus paragigantocellularis lateralis (von Euler, 1983). This structure is found ventro-laterally in the medulla oblongata, very close to the surface and just under the areas to which the central chemosensitivity has been localized. Focal cooling of the paragigantocellular nucleus elicits apnea (Cherniack et al, 1979 a). This structure mediates a successively increasing inspiratory activity during the inspiratory phase.

CENTRAL RESPIRATORY CONTROL

The chemoreceptor structures on the ventral medullary surface are responsible for the central carbon dioxide sensitivity. They react to the surrounding hydrogen ion concentration which reflects the carbon dioxide concentration in the blood. In these chemosensitive areas

Fukuda and Loeschcke (1977) have been able to record activity in superficial nerve cells which increase their firing rate when the surrounding hydrogen ion concentraton is increased, and vice versa. The usual mode of reaction of nerve cells is the opposite, i.e. inhibition when the surrounding pH is lowered.

By inhibiting central chemoreceptor activity by superfusion of the chemoreceptor areas with alkaline CSF it is possible to elicit periodic breathing in newborn rabbits and newborn guineapigs (Wennergren and Wennergren, 1980). Augmenting the oxygenation then by increasing the oxygen concentration in the inspired air normalized the breathing pattern as well as did increasing the carbon dioxide concentration in the inspired air (Wennergren and Wennergren 1983 a). In those experiments the mechanisms leading to periodic breathing could be the following. The superfusion with alkaline CSF reduces the respiratory drive from the central chemoreceptors. This withdrawal of an excitatory influence in combination with the central depressant effect of hypoxemia (Rigatto and Brady, 1972 b) due to the resulting diminished ventilation, leads to apnea. Progressive hyperapnia, combined with progressive hypoxemia, excites the peripheral chemoreceptors. The resulting respiratory drive leads to a sequence of breaths which improves oxygenation to a level where excitation of the peripheral chemoreceptors vanishes; a new short period of apnea resumes and so on (cf Lagercrantz et al, 1979). An increased oxygen concentration would here convert periodic breathing to steady by abolishing hypoxemia and removing its central depressant effect; the increased carbon dioxide concentration in the inspired would normalize periodic breathing by providing a continuous excitation of the peripheral and central chemoreceptors. The peripheral chemoreceptors have been considered to be a prerequisite for periodic breathing (Cherniack et al, 1979 b).

In a situation just after birth where the peripheral chemoreceptors not yet has been reset to operate at the higher PO_2-level present at extrauterine life (Blanco et al, 1984), a periodic breathing may be explained by a slowing down of the respiration when the respiratory centers are depressed by e.g. immaturity, sedation, few sensory stimuli or a low O_2 level. The PCO_2-level which then will rise will produce an increased respiratory drive via excitation of the central chemoreceptors. This will restitute respiration and increase the oxygen level while the PCO_2-level is successively lowered during increasing sensitivity to CO_2. The basicly low alertness of the respiratory center that was at hand and the diminishing CO_2 respiratory drive due to a transient overventilation leads again to a slowing down of the respiration. Initially the O_2 level decreases faster than the CO_2 level and a CO_2 accumulation with an increased respiratory drive is required for onset of a new accelerating breathing period.

The depressing influence of hypoxia has earlier been ascribed to a direct depressor action of hypoxia on the respiratory neurons but recent experiments by Dawes et al, (1983) suggest that action on specific structures in the brain stem above the pons level may convey the depressor effect of hypoxia.

Theophylline, which is used to counteract apneic spells in preterm babies has a marked excitatory effect on breathing when applied in small doses onto the ventral medullary surface. Spontaneously developing periodic breathing is promptly reversed to fast regular breathing by theophylline locally applied onto the ventral surface (Wennergren and Wennergren 1983). It seems reasonable to suggest that part of the stabilizing effect that theophylline has on irregular breathing is at the chemosensitive system, maybe at the nucleus paragigantocellularis lateralis where the central chemosensory signals converge (Loeschcke, 1980; Schlaefke, 1981). The mechanism by which theophylline acts could very well be by antagonizing endogenous adenosine. Endogenous adenosine is a potent inhibitor of synaptic transmission in the CNS and this action is blocked by the methyl-xanthines (Dunwiddie et al, 1981). Methylxanthines easily diffuse into CSF in the newborn infant (Somani et al, 1980). A leftward displacement of the CO_2-ventilation response curve, with (Davi et al, 1978) or without (Gerhardt et al, 1979) increased steepness of the curve, has been demonstrated in preterm infants treated with theophylline.

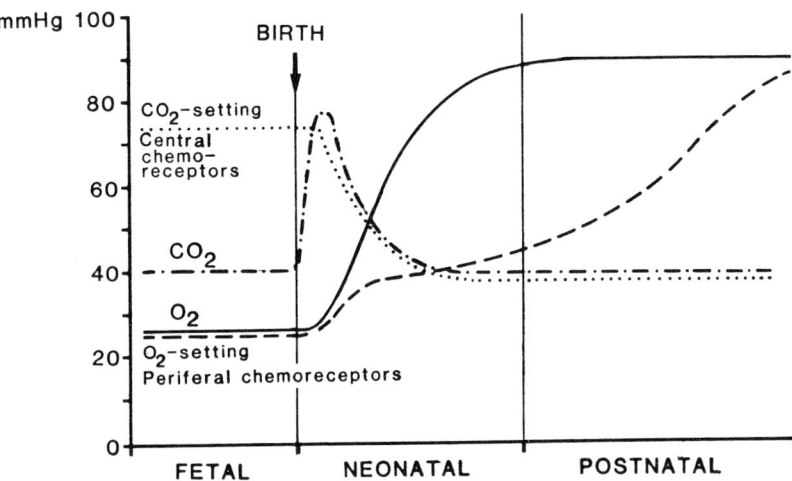

Fig. 6. The background for respiratory control mechanism around birth in a graphical model.

Pethidine (meperidine) applied topically onto the chemosensitive areas on the ventral medullary surface clearly inhibit breathing, an effect which is reversed by topically applied naloxone which also is the clinically used antidote (Wennergren and Wennergren, 1983 a). It is well known that pethidine decreases carbon dioxide sensitivity. It is probable that pethidine exerts at least part of its inhibitory influence, with delayed onset of breathing that can be seen at birth when the mother has been given pethidine, via an inhibition at the central chemosensitive system.

In experiments with exteriorized guinepig fetuses conversion of gasping or periodic breathing was seen just after superfusion of the central chemoreceptor zones with acid CSF had started (Wennergren and Wennergren, 1983 a). The observations are interesting and they support a view that the central chemoreceptors provide part of the respiratory drive that establishes a normal and regular respiration at birth.

RESPIRATORY CONTROL AROUND BIRTH

The respiratory control mechanisms around birth are scheduled in a graphical model in Fig. 6. The PO_2 level of 3-4 kPa before birth does not elicit breathing movements. This O_2 level is the normal living condition for growing, acting and functioning fetal cells. Thus for the fetus it is not 'considered' as hypoxia. Although peripheral chemoreceptors may react, their excitation does not 'reach through' and does not elicit breathing. The respiratory center in the medulla oblongata in other respects seems to be in a well functioning state, since at REM-sleep respiratory activity is relayed to the respiratory muscles.

The response threshold for CO_2 is set high in relation to fetal as well to extrauterine conditions, and does not take part in the control of the normal fetal condition.

After birth, before established breathing and with ceasing cord circulation, the disturbed gas exchange will cause a rapid development of respiratory acidosis and, with further lowered oxygen level, metabolic acidosis. The increasing biochemical stimuli 'go through', and a regular breathing is elicited. The O_2 level will rapidly exceed the fetal level, successively reaching 7-8 kPa or higher. There is obviously now a lowered response threshold for CO_2, with a rapid CO_2 blow off of CO_2 which reaches the earlier 'normal' level of 5.5 - 6 kPa.

Before the O_2 level starts to rise, there is as a rule a transient elevation of CO_2 which implies a respiratory excitation. Interpreted the other way around this indicates that an elevated O_2 plays a role by increasing responsiveness to CO_2.
However, at the same time there is a rich inflow of sensory stimuli, producing an increased CNS alertness. Since a lowered O_2 level during the neonatal period is followed by periodic breathing, it indicates that the O_2 level plays a role of its own in the control system. On the other hand, a reduction of sensory simuli may reduce the respiratory activity and reduce the CO_2 sensitivity. Taking also the rise of cathecholamine levels at birth into consideration there is the possibility for a variety of interactions between excitatory and inhibitory factors, allowing for a variation of patterns of onset of breathing. As negative factors may be added farmacological sedation and deep hypoxia preceeding birth as well as immaturity.

The adaptation to the higher extrauterine O_2 level with the peripheral chemoreceptors operating in the new oxygen range seems to take a certain time, at least through the neonatal period. During this adaptative period there may be risk for a 'reversed' reaction in relation to onset of breathing, eliciting apnea in preterm newborn infants with an immature respiratory center and instable lungaeration or pulmonary disorders. Such a 'reversed' reaction may also be a significant mechanism in the sudden infant death syndrome (cf Wennergren et al, 1983 b).

However, then the onset of breathing is passed long time ago.

ACKNOWLEDGEMENTS

We thank Ricardo Magno and Ingemar Kjellmer for generously giving us access to their original data, and Margareta Rydén for excellent typing of this manuscript.

REFERENCES

Blanco, C.E., Dawes, G.S., Hanson, M.A. & McCooke, H.B. (1984): The response to hypoxia of arterial chemoreceptors in fetal sheep and new-born lambs. J. Physiol. 351, 25-37.

Cherniack, N.S., Euler, C.v., Homma, I. & Kao, F.F. (1979 a): Graded changes in central chemoceptor input by local temperature changes on the ventral surface of medulla. J. Physiol. (Lond.) 287, 191-211.

Cherniack, N.S., Euler, C.v., Homma, I. & Kao, F.F. (1979 b): Experimentally induced Cheyne-Stokes breathing. Respir. Physiol. 37, 185-200.

Cross, K.W. & Oppé, T.E. (1952): The effect of inhalation of high and low concentrations of oxygen on the respiration of the premature infant. J. Physiol. (Lond.) 117, 38-55.

Davi, M.J., Sankaran, K., Simons, K.J., Simons, E.R., Seshia, M.M. & Rigatto, H. (1978): Physiologic changes induced by theophylline in the treatment of apnea in preterm infants. J. Pediatr. 92, 91-95.

Dawes, G.S., Fox, H.E., Leduc, B.M., G.C. & Richards, R.T. (1972): Respiratory movements and rapid eye movement sleep in the foetal lamb. J. Physiol. (Lond) 220, 119-143.

Dawes, G.S., Gardner, W.N., Johnstone, B.M. & Walker, D.W. (1983): Breathing in fetal lambs: the effect of brain stem section. J. Physiol. (Lond) 335, 535-553.

Dunwiddie, T.V., Hoffer, B.J. & Fredholm, B.B. (1981): Alkylxanthines elevate hippocampal excitability. Evidence for a role of endogenous adenosine. Naunyn-Schmiedeberg's Arch. Pharmacol. 316, 326-330.

Engström, I., Karlberg, P., Rooth, G., Tunell, R. (1966): The onset of respiration, a study of respiration and changes in blood gases and acid-base balance. Association for the Aid of Crippled Children, New York.

Euler, C. von. (1983): On the central pattern generator for the basic breathing rhytmicity. J. Appl. Physiol.: Respirat. Environ. Exercise Physiol. 55, 1647-1659.

Euler, C. von. (1985): Brain-stem mechanisms for generation and control of the breathing pattern. In: Handbook of Physiology. The respiratory system. Bethseda: Am. Physiol. Soc., sect 3, vol II. In press.

Fukuda, Y. & Loescheke, H.H. (1977): Effect of H^+ on spontaneous neuronal activity in the surface layer of the rat medulla oblongata in vitro. Pfluegers Arch. 371, 125-134.

Gerhardt, T., McCarty, J. & Bancalari, E. (1979): Effect of aminophylline on respiratory center activity and metabolic rate in premature infants with idiopathic apnea. Pediatrics 63, 537-542.

Gluckman, P.D., Gunn, T.R. & Johnstone, B.M. (1983): The effect of cooling on breathing and shivering in unanesthetized fetal lambs in utero. J. Physiol. 343, 495-506.

Grögaard, J., Lindstrom, D.P., Stahlman, M., Marchal, F. & Sundell, H. (1982): The cardiovascular response to laryngeal water administration in young lambs. J. Dev. Physiol. 4, 353-370.

Grögaard, J. & Sundell, H. (1983): Effect of Beta-Adrenergic Agonists on Apnea Reflexes in Newborn Lambs. Ped. Res. 17, 213-219.

Karlberg, P. (1958): Breathing and its control in premature infants. In: Physiology of Prematurity, (ed): Transactions of the Second Conference, March 25, 26 and 27 1957, ed J.Y. Lanman, p 77. Madison, New Jersey: Madison Printing Company, Inc.

Karlberg, P. (1960): The adaptive changes in the immediate postnatal period, with particular reference to respiration. The Journ. of Pediatr. 56, 585-604.

Karlberg, P. Cherry, R.B., Escardo, F. & Koch, G. (1962): Respiratory studies in newborn infants. II. Pulmonary centilation and mechanics of breathing in the first minutes of life, including the onset of respiration. Acta Paediatr. Scand. 51, 121-136.

Karlberg, P. & Celander, O. (1965 a): Respiratory and circulatory adaptation in the newborn infant with particular reference to the immediate postnatal period. In Recent Advances of Paediatrics, 3rd edn, ed D. Gaidner, pp 36-53.

Karlberg, P., Moore, R.E. & Oliver, T.K. Jr. (1965 b): Thermogenic and cardiovascular responses of the newborn baby to noradrenaline. Acta Paediatr. Scand. 54, 225-238.

Karlberg, P. (1985): Onset of breathing. In The Roots of Perinatal Medicine, ed G. Rooth, O.D. Saugstad, pp 76-85. Stuttgart: Georg Thieme.

Kjellmer, I., Magno, R. & Karlsson, K. (1974): Anesthesia for cesarean section. I: Effects on the respiratory adaptation of the newborn in elective cesarean section. Acta Anesth. Scand. 18, 48-57.

Lagercrantz, H. & Bistoletti, P. (1977): Catecholamine release in the newborn infant at birth. Ped. Res. 11, 889-893.

Lagercrantz, H., Ahlström, H., Jonson, B., Lindroth, M. & Svenningsen, N. (1979): A critical oxygen level below which irregular breathing occurs in preterm infants. In: Central nervous control mechanisms in breathing (ed C.v. Euler & H. Lagercrantz). Wenner-Gren Center International Symposium Series, vol. 32, pp. 161-164.

Loeschcke, H.H. (1980): Chemical alterations of cerebrospinal fluid acting on respiratory and circulatory control systems. In: Neurobiology of cerebrospinal fluid 1, ed J. H. Wood, pp 29-40. New York: Plenum Press.

Magno, R., Selstam, U. & Karlsson, K. (1975): Anesthesia for cesarean section. II: Effects of the Induction - Delivery interval on the respiratory adaptation of the newborn in elective cesarean section. Acta Anesth. Scand. 19, 250-259.

Magno. R., Kjellmer, I. & Karlsson, K. (1976 a): Anesthesia for cesarean section. III: Effects of epidural analgesia on the respiratory adaptation of the newborn in elective cesarean section. Acta Anesth. Scand. 20, 73-82.

Magno, R., Karlsson, K., Selstam, U. & Wickström, I. (1976 b): Anesthesia for cesarean section. V: Effects of enflurane anesthesia on the respiratory adaptation of the newborn in elective cesarean section. Acta Anesth. Scand. 20, 147-155.

Rigatto, H. & Brady, J.P. (1972 a): Periodic breathing and apnea in preterm infants. I. Evidence for hypoventilation possibly due to central respiratory depression. Pediatrics 50, 202-218.

Rigatto, H. & Brady, J.P. (1972 b): Periodic breathing and apnea in preterm infants. II. Hypoxia as a primary event. Pediatrics 50, 219-228.

Schlaefke, M.E. (1981): Central chemosensitivity: a respiratory drive. Rev. Physiol. Biochem. Pharmacol. 90, 171-244.

Somani, S.M., Khanna, N.N. & Bada, H.S. (1980): Caffeine and theophylline: serum/CSF correlation in premature infants. J. Pediatr. 96, 1091-1093.

Tunell, R., Copher, D. & Persson, B. (1976): Pulmonary gas exchange and blood gas changes in connection with birth. In Neonatal Intensive Care, eds J.B. Stetson, P.R. Swyer, p 89. St Louis: Warren H. Green.

Walters. D.V. & Olver, R.E. (1978): The role of cathecholamines in lung liquid absorption at birth. Pediatr. Res. 12, 239-242.

Wennergren, G. & Wennergren, M. (1980): Respiratory effects elicited in newborn animals via the central chemoreceptors. Acta Physiol. Scand. 108, 309-311.

Wennergren, G. & Wennergren, M. (1983 a): Neonatal breathing control mediated via the central chemoreceptors. Acta Physiol. Scand. 119, 139-146.

Wennergren, G., Bjure, J. & Kjellmer, I. (1983 b): A case of near-miss sids developing an abnormal respiratory reaction to hypoxia. Acta Paediatr, Scand. 72, 793-795.

Wennergren, M., Krantz, M., Hjalmarson, O. & Karlsson, K. (1985): Time from rupture of membranes to delivery and its influence upon neonatal respiratory diseases. In 2nd International symposium on "The fetus as a patient, diagnosis and therapy". Abstracts. Jerusalem: Abstr. 144.

RESUME

L'adaptation à la vie extra-utérine implique des modifications drastiques sur le plan fonctionnel, dont la pierre angulaire est la mise en route de la respiration aérienne. Les mécanismes de contrôle de cette respiration sont différents de ceux qui régulaient les mouvements respiratoires foetaux.

Dans les 10-20 secondes après la naissance, le nouveau-né accomplit sa première respiration, de grande amplitude, suivie de cycles généralement irréguliers entrecoupés de pauses, mais laissant vite place à une respiration régulière. Les échanges gazeux commencent dès la première minute et la perfusion sanguine pulmonaire augmente rapidement. Dans des conditions normales, la respiration est bien établie en 10 à 20 minutes.

Le point de départ, i.e. la situation foetale, est résumé sur la figure 2.

Les stimuli et la séquence biochimique sont alors les suivants: avant le démarrage de la respiration, la PCO_2 s'élève, la PO_2 chute et il s'installe une acidose à la fois respiratoire et métabolique; ceci persiste jusqu'à ce qu'une respiration régulière soit établie. L'association de l'hypercapnie, de l'hypoxie, et de l'acidose, stimule les chémorécepteurs périphériques. Ceux-ci n'ont pas encore été réajustés au nouveau seuil de réglage ("point de consigne") approprié aux PO_2 élevées régnant à l'air libre: des stimuli biochimiques suffisamment forts réussissent cependant à les mettre en jeu. Quand l'oxygénation s'améliore, la PCO_2 descend se stabiliser autour de ˹ kPa et l'acidose métabolique disparait lentement.

Les stimuli sensoriels s'abattent en foule sur le nouveau-né: visuels, tactiles, thermiques surtout (importance primordiale des récepteurs au froid, l'immersion en bain chaud pouvant bloquer la respiration).

La montée des catécholamines pendant le travail s'accompagne d'une réactivité accrue du nouveau-né qui facilite la respiration; par ailleurs la stimulation des béta-récepteurs déclenche l'arrêt de la production du liquide pulmonaire, aidant ainsi à l'adaptation respiratoire.

Les structures nerveuses responsables du contrôle respiratoire réalisent essentiellement des variations rythmées de l'activité inspiratoire, à partir d'un groupe dorsal et d'un groupe ventral de neurones situés dans le bulbe. Les neurones inspiratoires doivent garder in tonus de base, maintenu pendant la veille par les stimuli sensoriels et pendant le sommeil par les afférences des chémorécepteurs périphériques et centraux.

Les chémorécepteurs bulbaires ventraux sont responsables de la sensibilité au CO_2. Pendant la respiration périodique spontanée, l'application locale de théophylline dans cette zone réinstalle rapidement une respiration régulière (possible effet antagoniste de l'adénosine endogène). Par contre, l'application de péthidine dans la même zone inhibe la respiration, effet aboli par l'application de naloxone.

La figure 6 résume les mécanismes de contrôle mis en jeu à la naissance. Le seuil de réponse au CO2 s'abaisse. L'adaptation au niveau supérieur de PO2 caractérisant la vie extra-utérine exige un certain temps.

Il y a donc de nombreuses interactions entre les facteurs stimulants et les facteurs inhibiteurs, et chaque cas de figure peut engendrer un type différent de mise en route de la respiration aérienne.

———

Respiratory adaptation and hormonal surge at birth: possible sex differences

G. Faxelius, K. Bremme*, H. Lagercrantz and J. Milerad

*Departments of Paediatrics and *Obstetrics and Gynaecology, Karolinska Hospital, Karolinska Institute, Stockholm, Sweden*

ABSTRACT

Sex differences in the incidence of hyaline membrane disease (HMD) after vaginal delivery vs caesarean section were investigated in 159 preterm infants ≤ 34 weeks gestation. After vaginal delivery the HMD incidence was 33.3 percent in the male and 6.5 percent in the female infants (p < 0.005), whereas after caesarean section the incidence was the same when comparing males and females. In female infants the HMD occurrence was considerably lower (p < 0.001) after vaginal delivery (6.5 percent) than after caesarean section (42.8 percent). In order to relate the sex differences in respiratory adaptation after vaginal delivery vs caesarean section to hormonal surge, plasma levels of catecholamines, cortisol, and prolactin were measured at birth in term neonates. However, no significant differences in hormonal levels between male and female infants were found. The findings suggest that female in contrast to male preterm infants respond to the stress of labor by accelerated pulmonary maturity.

KEY WORDS

Newborn, premature, hyaline membrane disease, caesarean section, catecholamines, sex

CATECHOLAMINE AND CORTICOSTEROID SURGE AT BIRTH

During vaginal delivery there is a general surge of hormones such as corticosteroids (Ohrlander et al, 1976; Talbert et al, 1977) and catecholamines (Lagercrantz & Bistoletti, 1977; Irestedt et al, 1982). Considerably lower levels of cortisol and catecholamines were found after elective caesarean section. This hormonal surge is important for the neonatal respiratory adaptation. In studies on fetal sheep, adrenaline has been found to inhibit lung liquid secretion and even stimulate its absorption (Walters & Olver, 1978). Adrenaline is also known to stimulate surfactant release (Lawson et al, 1978). Glucorticocoids stimulate synthesis of surfactant (Ballard et al, 1977; Liggins & Howie, 1972) and enhance the effects of the sympathoadrenal system in increasing pulmonary beta-adrenergic receptors (Cheng et al, 1980).

HORMONAL SURGE AND RESPIRATORY ADAPTATION

The possible importance of the increased sympatho-adrenal activity at birth for the respiratory adaptation of the neonate was previously studied (Faxelius et al, 1983). Lung function was measured at 30 minutes and two hours after birth in two groups of healthy neonates, one delivered vaginally and one delivered by elective caesarean

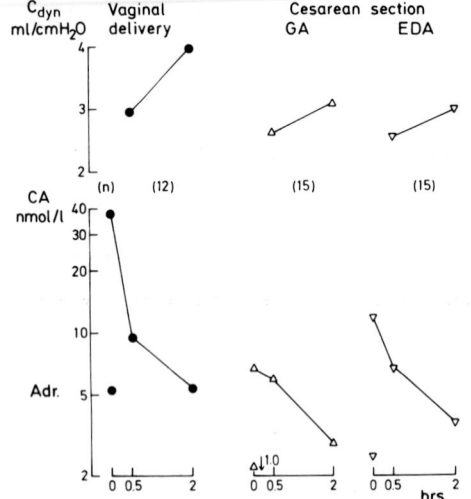

Fig. 1. Dynamic lung compliance (C dyn), catecholamine (CA), and adrenaline (Adr) levels in term infants after vaginal delivery vs caesarean section under general (GA) and epidural (EDA) anaesthesia (mean values). The difference in C dyn was significant at two hours between vaginal and the caesarean section groups ($p < 0.01$).

section. Catecholamines and cortisol were measured at birth and showed significantly higher levels in infants delivered vaginally. Dynamic lung compliance was similar in the two types of deliveries at 30 minutes, but increased significantly more in the vaginally delivered group than in the caesarean section group at two hours (Fig. 1). Furthermore, a significant correlation was found ($r = 0.84$) between the catecholamine concentrations at birth and dynamic lung compliance. The results indicate a delayed clearance of lung liquid in the infants delivered by caesarean section with the lower catecholamine levles as a contributing factor. Our observation of an impaired lung function within the first few hours after birth in infants delivered by elective caesarean section is supported by previous reports (Milner et al, 1978; Boon et al, 1981).

Infants delivered by caesarean section often have respiratory disorders of various degree after birth, e.g., transient tachypnea (Hjalmarson et al, 1982) and hyaline membrane disease (HMD) in case of prematurity (Usher et al, 1971; Fedrick & Butler, 1972). This was further confirmed in a previous retrospective study on the incidence of HMD and type of delivery (Faxelius et al, 1982). The occurrence of HMD was found to be significantly higher after caesarean section but only beyond 34 weeks gestation.

SEX DIFFERENCE

The incidence and severity of HMD is increased in male infants as reported in several studies (Miller & Futrakul, 1968; Papageorgiou et al, 1981). Furthermore, antenatal corticosteroid therapy for prevention of HMD is less effective in male than in female infants (Ballard et al, 1980; Papageorgiou et al, 1981). In reviewing the above mentioned study (Faxelius et al, 1982) on HMD incidence in 159 infants ≤ 34 weeks gestation a considerably higher occurrence of HMD was found in male than in female infants, 37.6 vs 20.2 percent. After vaginal delivery the incidence of HMD was 6.5 percent in the female and 33.3 percent in the male infant, whereas no difference existed after caesarean section. In the female infants the HMD occurrence was significantly reduced after vaginal delivery (6.5 percent) when compared to the incidence after caesarean section (42.8 percent) in contrast to the male infants, in whom no influence on HMD incidence by mode of delivery was evident (Fig. 2). No important differences in birth weight or gestational age were found between male and female infants in the two delivery groups (Table 1).

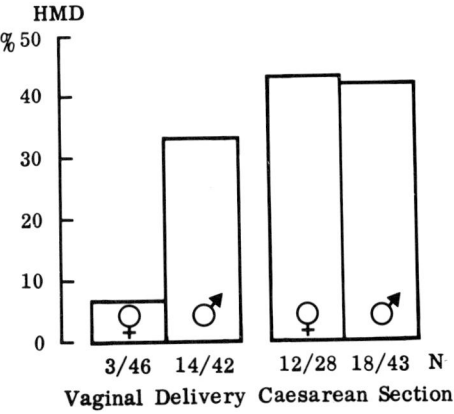

Fig. 2. Incidence of hyaline membrane disease (HMD) in male and female infants ≤ 34 weeks gestation delivered by caesarean section and vaginally. The difference was significant between females and males delivered vaginally ($p < 0.005$) and between female infants delivered vaginally and by caesarean section ($p < 0.001$).

Table 1. Birth weight and gestational age in male and female infants ≤ 34 weeks gestation delivered vaginally and by caesarean section (mean values ± 1 SD).

	Vaginal delivery		Caesarean section	
	males n = 42	females n = 46	males n = 43	females n = 28
Gestational age, weeks	30.3 ± 2.2	30.7 ± 2.5	31.5 ± 1.9	32.3 ± 1.6
Birth weight, g	1385 ± 332	1384 ± 352	1510 ± 316	1528 ± 279

The findings support previous reports (Miller & Futrakul, 1968; Papageorgiou et al, 1981) on increased incidence of HMD in male infants and suggest that female in contrast to male preterm infants below 35 weeks gestation respond to the stress of labour by accelerated pulmonary maturity as evidenced by the lower incidence of HMD in female infants after vaginal delivery when compared to caesarean section. One explanation is a sex difference in surfactant production, with lower surfactants produced in males, which has been demonstrated both in clinical (Torday et al, 1981) and animal studies (Nielsen & Torday, 1981). The lag of surfactant production observed in the male preterm infant has been suggested to be due to an inhibition of fetal surfactant production by fetal circulating androgen (Nielsen et al, 1982). Differences in levels of hormones important for surfactant synthesis such as cortisol (Ballard et al, 1977; Liggins & Howie, 1972) and prolactin (Hamosh & Hamosh, 1977) might be another contributing factor to the differences in pulmonary maturity between male and female infants. Higher levels of cortisol in amniotic fluid (Torday et al, 1981) and of prolactin in cord blood (Dhanireddy et al, 1983) were observed in female preterm infants than were observed in male preterm infants.

CATECHOLAMINES, CORTICOSTEROIDS, AND PROLACTIN CONCENTRATIONS
IN NEWBORN BOYS AND GIRLS

Differences in sympatho-adrenal activity and in maturity of the beta-adrenergic receptors in the lung is another possible explanation. Adrenaline inhibits lung liquid secretion (Walters & Olver, 1978) and promotes surfactant release (Lawson et al, 1978). Furthermore, antenatal treatment of beta-adrenergic agonists to prevent preterm labour seems to lead to a decreased incidence of HMD (Bergman & Hedner, 1978). A delay in lung beta-adrenergic receptors and adrenal medullary maturation has been demonstrated in male rabbit fetuses (Padbury et al, 1981).

Table 2. Plasma noradrenaline, adrenaline, cortisol, and prolactin concentrations at birth (umbilical artery) in term male and female infants delivered vaginally and by caesarean section (median values and range).

	Vaginal delivery			Caesarean section		
	males	females	p*	males	females	p*
Noradrenaline, nmol/l						
median	31.4	19.5	0.058	8.7	4.9	ns
range	9.9-132.3	3.7-70.4		1.7-16.9	1.7-23.2	
n	30	20		15	12	
Adrenaline, nmol/l						
median	3.9	3.1	0.078	1.7	0.8	0.086
range	0.01-23.1	0.01-13.5		0.2-5.9	0.01-3.9	
n	28	20		15	12	
Cortisol, nmol/l						
median	438	527	ns	300	245	ns
range	130-966	289-1308		83-828	77-795	
n	21	11		10	9	
Prolactin, nmol/l						
median	263	265	ns	220		ns
range	76-576	111-460		76-360		
n	19	8		7		

* Mann-Whitney rank sum test was used.

To test possible sex differences in sympatho-adrenal activity, plasma levels of noradrenaline and adrenaline were analysed from umbilical arterial blood at birth as previously described (Irestedt et al, 1982) in healthy full-term neonates delivered vaginally or by elective caesarean section. Levels of cortisol and prolactin were liekwise measured. Infants with umbilical pH below 7.22 were excluded. No important differences in Apgar scores, umbilical arterial pH, birth weight, or gestational age were found between the male and female infants in the two delivery groups.

Although the male infants seemed to have higher levels or noradrenaline and adrenaline the difference proved not to be statistically significant. Previous reports on both term (Padbury et al, 1982) and preterm (Newnham et al, 1984) fetuses likewise showed no significant differences in catecholamine levels in the two sexes. However, considerably higher urine catecholamine levels were found in male than in female infants from the first day to $3\frac{1}{2}$ months of life (Dahlmaz & Peyrin, 1982).

No sex-related differences in cortisol or prolactin levels in our study were observed. As in previous studies (Lagercrantz & Bistoletti, 1977; Irestedt et al, 1982), significant higher levels of catecholamines and cortisol were found after vaginal delivery.

CONCLUSIONS

The hormonal surge during labour is important for the respiratory adaptation of the neonate as proven by enhanced respiratory performance and good correlation between catecholamines and dynamic lung compliance in the first few hours after birth in vaginally delivered infants. This is further supported by the clinical observation of increased occurrence of HMD in preterm infants after caesarean section. The incidence of HMD is increased in male preterm infants below 35 weeks gestation and is not influenced by mode of delivery. In the female preterm infants a considerably lower HMD incidence after vaginal delivery than after caesarean section indicates an accelerated pulmonary maturity when compared to the male infants and also gives further evidence for the important role that labour has in regard to respiratory adaptation. Plasma levels of catecholamines, cortisol, and prolactin in term neonates at birth did not show any sex-related differences to explain a delay in pulmonary maturity in male infants. Sex differences in the maturity of the pulmonary beta-adrenergic receptors need to be further investigated.

ACKNOWLEDGEMENTS

We thank Mrs Ingrid Dahlin for technical assistance. This study was supported by grant no. 5234 from the Swedish Medical Research Council, and Sällskapet Barnavård.

REFERENCES

Ballard, P.L., Benson, B.J. & Brehier, A. (1977): Glucocorticoid effects in the fetal lung. Am. Rev. Respir. Dis. 115, 29-36.
Ballard, P.L., Ballard, R.A., Granberg, P.J., Sniderman, S., Gluckman, P.D., Kaplan, S.L. & Grumbach, M.M. (1980): Fetal sex and prenatal betamethasone therapy. J. Pediatr. 97, 451-454.
Bergman, B. & Hedner, T. (1978): Antepartum administration of terbutaline and the incidence of hyaline membrane disease in preterm infants. Acta Obstet. Gynecol. Scand. 57, 285-288.
Bistoletti, P., Nylund, L., Lagercrantz, H., Hjemdahl, P. & Ström, H. (1983): Fetal scalp catecholamines during labor. Am. J. Obstet. Gyencol. 147, 785-788.
Boon, A.W., Milner, A.D. & Hopkins, I.F. (1981): Lung volumes and lung mechanics in babies born vaginally and by elective and emergency lower segmental caesarean section. J. Pediatr. 98, 812-815.
Cheng, J.B., Goldfein, A., Ballard, P.L. & Roberts, J.M. (1980): Glucocorticoids increase pulmonary beta-adrenergic receptors in fetal rabbit. Endocrinology 107, 1646-1648.
Dahlmaz, Y. & Peyrin, L. (1982): Sex-differences in catecholamine metabolites in human urine during development and at adulthood. J. Neurol. Transm. 54, 193-207.
Dhanireddy, R., Smith, Y.F., Hamosh, M., Mullon, J.W., Scanlon, J.W. & Hamosh, P. (1983): Respiratory distress syndrome in the newborn: Relationship to serum prolactin, thyroxine, and sex. Biol. Neonate 43, 9-15.
Faxelius, G., Bremme, K. & Lagercrantz, H. (1982): An old problem revisited – Hyaline membrane disease and cesarean section. Eur. J. Pediatr. 139, 121-124.
Faxelius, G., Hägnevik, K., Lagercrantz, H., Lundell, B. & Irestedt, L. (1983): Catecholemine surge and lung function after delivery. Arch. Dis. Child. 58, 262-266.
Fedrick, J. & Butler, N.R. (1972): Hyaline membrane disease. Lancet 2, 768-769.
Hamosh, M & Hamosh, P. (1977): The effect of prolactin on the lecithin content of fetal rabbit lung. J. Clin. Invest. 59, 1002-1005.
Hjalmarson, O., Krantz, M.E., Jakobsson, B. & Sörensen, S.E. (1982): The importance of neonatal asphyxia and caesarean section as risk factors for neonatal respiratory disorders. Acta Paediatr, Scand. 71, 403-408.
Irestedt, L., Lagercrantz, H., Hjemdahl, P., Hägnevik, K. & Belfrage, P. (1982): Fetal and maternal plasma catecholamine levels at elective cesarean section under general or epidural anesthesia versus vaginal delivery. Am. J. Obstet. Gynecol. 142, 1004-1010.
Lagercrantz, H & Bistoletti, P. (1977): Catecholamine release in the newborn infant at birth. Pediatr. Res 11. 889-893.

Lawson, B.B., Brown, E.R., Torday, J.S., Madansky, D.L. & Taeusch, W.H. (1978): The effect of epinephrine on tracheal fluid flow and surfactant efflux in fetal sheep. Am. Rev. Respir. Dis. 118, 1023-1026.

Liggins, G.C. & Howie, R.N. (1972): A controlled trial of antepartum glucocorticoid treatment for prevention of respiratory distress syndrome in premature infants. Pediatrics 50, 515-525.

Miller, H.C. & Futrakul, P. (1968): Birthweight, gestational age, and sex as determining factors in the incidence of respiratory distress syndrome of prematurly born infants. J. Pediatr. 72, 628-635.

Milner, A.D., Saunders, R.A. & Hopkins, I.E. (1978): Effects of delivery by caesarean section on lung mechanics and lung volume in the human neonate. Arch. Dis. Child. 53, 545-548.

Newnham, J.P., Marshall, C.L., Padbury, J.F., Lam, R.W., Hobel, C.J. & Fisher, D.A. (1984): Fetal catecholamine release with preterm delivery. Am. J. Obstet. Gyencol. 149, 888-893.

Nielsen, H.C. & Torday, J.S. (1981): Sex differences in fetal rabbit pulmonary surfactant production. Pediatr. Res. 15, 1245-1247.

Nielsen, H.C., Zinman, H.M. & Torday, J.S. (1982): Dihydrotestosterone inhibits fetal rabbit pulmonary surfactant production. J. Clin. Invest 69, 611-616.

Ohrlander, S., Gennser, G. & Eneroth, P. (1976): Plasma cortisol levels in human fetus during parturition. Obstet. Gynecol. 48, 381-387.

Padbury, J.F., Hobel, C.J., Lam, R.W. & Fisher, P.A. (1981): Sex differences in lung and adrenal neurosympathetic development in rabbits. Am. J. Obstet. Gyencol. 1941, 199-204.

Padbury, J.F., Roberman, B., Oddie, T.H., Hobel, C.J. & Fisher, D.A. (1982): Fetal catecholamine release in response to labor and delivery. Obstet. Gynecol. 60, 607-611.

Papageorgiou, A.N., Colle, E., Farri-Kostopoulos, E. & Gelfland, M.M. (1981): Incidence of respiratory distress syndrome following antenatal betamethasone: Role of sex, type of delivery and prolonged rupture of membranes. Pediatrics 67:614-617.

Talbert, L.M., Pearlman, W.H. & Potter, D.M. (1977): Maternal and fetal serum levels of total cortisol and cortisone, unbound cortisol and corticosteroid-binding globulin in vaginal delivery and cesarean section. Am. J. Obstet. Gynecol 129, 781-787.

Torday, J.S., Nielsen, H.C., de Fencl, M. & Avery, M.E. (1981): Sex differences in fetal lung maturation. Am. Rev. Respir. Dis. 123, 205-208.

Usher, R.H., Allen, A.C. & McLean, F.H. (1971): Risk of respiratory distress syndrome related to gestational age, route of delivery and maternal diabetes. Am. J. Obstet. Gynecol. 111, 826-832.

Walters, D.V. & Olver, R.E. (1978): The role of catecholamines in lung liquid absorption at birth. Pediatr. Res. 12, 239-242.

Wurtman, R.J. & Axelrod, J. (1966): Control of enzymatic synthesis of adrenaline in the adrenal medulla by adrenal cortical steroids. J. Biol. Chem. 241, 2301-2305.

RESUME

Après naissance par voie basse, il se produit chez le nouveau-né une montée des taux de corticostéroides et de catécholamines, alors que ces taux restent beaucoup plus faibles après naissance par césarienne. Cette poussée hormonale joue un rôle important dans l'adaptation respiratoire néonatale.

Une étude précédente (Faxelius et al., 1983) avait montré l'importance possible de l'augmentation d'activité sympatho-surrénale à la naissance: la fonction respiratoire (compliance dynamique) était évaluée à 30 minutes et à 2 heures après la naissance dans 2 groupes de nouveau-nés sains, un groupe d'enfants nés par voie basse et un groupe d'enfants nés par césarienne élective. Les résultats montraient un retard d'élimination de liquide pulmonaire chez les enfants nés par césarienne, en association avec de plus faibles taux de catécholamines.

La fréquence de troubles respiratoires de diverse gravité a été trouvée plus élevée après naissance par césarienne, en particulier le taux de maladie des membranes hyalines (MMH)(Faxelius et al., 1982). Cette même étude avait aussi noté une fréquence beaucoup plus élevée de MMH chez les garçons que chez les filles (37,6 pour cent contre 20,2 pour cent): en réalité, il n'existait pas de différence selon le sexe après naissance par césarienne, mais chez les filles le taux de MMH était de 6,5 pour cent après voie basse contre 42,8 pour cent après césarienne. Il n'y avait pas de différences significatives de poids de naissance ni d'âge gestationnel entre les groupes. Ces résultats en accord avec d'autres publications font penser que les foetus de sexe féminin au-dessous de 35 semaines réagissent au stress du travail en accélérant leur maturation pulmonaire (la production de surfactant est donc moindre chez les garçons). En plus des taux supérieurs de cortisol dans le liquide amniotique et de prolactine dans le sang du cordon observés chez les filles, une autre explication de cette différence de maturation pulmonaire pourrait résider dans les variations de l'activité sympatho-surrénale et de la maturité des récepteurs béta-adrénergiques pulmonaires selon le sexe. Dans le sang artériel prélevé au cordon chez des nouveau-nés sains, les taux plasmatiques de nor-adrénaline et d'adrénaline étaient légèrement supérieurs chez les garçons mais la différence n'était pas significative. Les taux plasmatiques de cortisol et de prolactine étaient très similaires dans les 2 groupes (Tableau 2).

En Conclusion, les taux plasmatiques de catécholamines, cortisol, et prolactine chez le nouveau-né à terme ne diffèrent pas selon le sexe et n'expliquent pas le retard de maturation pulmonaire des garçons. Il est donc nécessaire de poursuivre les recherches en direction de possibles différences de maturation des récepteurs béta-adrénergiques pulmonaires.

****

DISCUSSION. Dr.W.Oh, moderator.

Dr.J.Warshaw: A possible explanation to catechol receptor defects would be that boys are intrinsically less mature and have a decrease in the available surfactant pool. Nielsen, in our department, has looked at this dimorphism in experimental animals: the TF mouse, which is a mouse model with testicular feminization due to the absence of cytoplasmic receptors for androgens, shows normal lung development whereas normal males are delayed (Amer.Rev.Resp.Dis. 1984; 129:294A). This effect is likely due to a direct link between the process controlling sex differentiation and lung maturation.

Pr.P.Karlberg: We know that girls are ahead of boys; the only thing in which they are equal is eruption of the deciduous teeth. I have two comments. The first deals with catecholamine production during labour and delivery. In our department, in one year of total perinatal population of 4500 deliveries, all neonates were carefully followed according to respiratory disturbances. When C-section was performed after labor had started or after premature rupture of membranes, the full-term newborn infants showed a lower incidence of respiratory disturbances than the ones born by elective C-section. (Unpublished data, Hjalmarson et al.). My second comment refers to dynamic compliance after vaginal deliveries. May the difference in limb circulation indicate a redistribution of blood flow, which then influences the lung elasticity?

Dr.G.Faxelius: It might mean that there is an increased pulmonary blood flow which would also facilitate the pulmonary adaptation.

Dr.W.Oh: Can you tell us what was the distribution of birthweights between the 2 sexes within the group of less than 34 weeks babies? When dealing with HMD, 34-33-32 week-old babies fare generally well but below 32 weeks of gestation, the picture is very different. I wonder what the difference was for weights in boys versus girls belo below 32 weeks?

Dr.G.Faxelius: There was no important difference in birthweights or gestational age between boys and girls, as shown in Table 1 (see the above paper).

Dr.L.Stern: The differences you showed were essentially in noradrenaline levels. Catecholamine proportions in neonates comprise mostly noradrenaline and very little adrenaline. I wonder how reliable are the differences in epinephrine because the quantities should be very small?

Dr.H.Lagercrantz: With the HPLC method, you can easily differentiate between noradrenaline and adrenaline. With the old fluorination method, it was much more difficult, particularly when the noradrenaline:adrenaline ration was very high as in the newborn infant (about 7:1).

Dr.J.Metcoff: Were there any differences in the occurrence of transient tachypnea?

Dr.G.Faxelius: We did not look into that.

Dr.W.Oh: It is often difficult to separate out which respiratory distress cases are due to fluid problems and which are due to surfactant; to attribute the differences to hormonal changes is quastionable.

Dr.H.Lagercrantz: The difference in RDS between vaginally versus C-section delivered infants was most remarkable in the full-term infants, indicating that the fluid problem was the most important.

Adenosine—a neuromodulator released during asphyxia and a mediator of some hypoxic effects in the newborn?

H. Lagercrantz, B.B. Fredholm, L. Irestedt, M. Runold and A. Sollevi

Nobel Institute for Neurophysiology, Department of Pharmacology, Karolinska Institute and Department of Pediatrics and Anaesthesiology, Karolinska Hospital, S 104 01 Stockholm, Sweden

ABSTRACT

Adenosine release is markedly increased during delivery particularly after asphyxia, as indicated by high concentrations of the adenosine metabolite hypoxanthine in cord blood. A stable adenosine analogue, L-N^6-phenyl-isopropyl-adenosine (PIA), was found to strongly depress ventilation, particularly in the youngest animals and cause sedation, hypotonia and hypothermia, in rabbit pups.

Adenosine released during asphyxia in the newborn might be responsible for some of the symptoms seen after perinatal asphyxia. Furthermore adenosine might counteract the effects of catecholamines, which also are released during perinatal asphyxia.

KEY WORDS

Adenosine, perinatal asphyxia, apnoea, hypothermia, catecholamines.

During perinatal asphyxia and particularly at the moment of birth there is a surge of neurohormones e.g. catecholamines (Lagercrantz & Bistoletti 1977), vasopressin (Pohjavuori & Fyhrquist 1980) and endorphins (Wardlaw et al. 1979). Also adenosine is probably released in high concentrations during perinatal asphyxia as indicated by high fetal concentrations of hypoxanthine (Saugstad 1975). Already 1929 Drury & Szent-Györgyi reported that adenosine was found to depress ventilation and cause sedation and hypotension in the adult cat and adenosine is then one of the first described neuromodulators. The recent interest is due to the finding that adenosine, which is released during cerebral hypoxia (Winn, Rubio & Berne 1981), might mediate a number of hypoxic effects causing vasodilatation both in the systemic and cerebral circulation, sedation, hypothermia, inhibit lipolysis and glycogenolysis (Burnstock 1981) and depress the respiration (Hedner et al. 1982; Lagercrantz et al. 1984; Eldridge et al. 1984).

Specific receptors for adenosine exist and theophylline may exert some of its therapeutic effects e.g. its preventive action on recurrent apnoea in preterm infants, by blockade of adenosine receptors (c.f. Fredholm 1982).

In this article we consider the role of adenosine as a chemical mediator of some hypoxic effects in the newborn. The hypothesis is that a number of symptoms seen in the asphyxiated newborn infant might be partially attributed to endogenously released adenosine. Obviously other neurohormones such as the endorphins are also released during perinatal asphyxia (Wardlaw et al. 1979) and to some extent they have similar actions as adenosine. Probably the newborn is provided with several neurohormonal systems acting in concert during stress.

ORIGIN OF ADENOSINE

Adenosine is formed everywhere adenine nucleotides are split like in the muscles, blood corpuscles, platelets, reticuloendothelial system and glia cells. ATP has been proposed to be a neurotransmitter in purinergic nerves, particularly in the intestines (Burnstock 1981). Furthermore, ATP is a co-transmitter, stored together with catecholamines in the ratio of 1:4 in the adrenal medulla and in a lower ratio together with noradrenaline in sympathetic neurons and in cholinergic nerves (see Klein, Lagercrantz & Zimmerman 1982). It is possible that purinergic neurons appear early ontogenetically and it has been shown that the ATP:catecholamine ratio is higher in the fetal adrenal medulla than in the adult one.

Adenosine is thus released as a consequence of increased metabolic and neural activity (Phillis & Wu 1981). Furthermore it is released during hypoxia in various organs including the brain. Winn et al (1981) have clearly demonstrated that the concentration of adenosine is considerably increased during hypoxia; when the arterial PO_2 was lowered to 30 mm Hg during five minutes in the adult rat there was a seven-fold increase of the adenosine concentration in the whole brain.

Adenosine has as far as we know not been determined in severely asphyxiated infants, but a number of studies on measurement of the adenosine metabolite hypoxanthine in umbilical blood have been published (Saugstad 1975; Thiringer 1982). These studies have demonstrated that there is a relationship between the degree of asphyxia and hypoxanthine concentrations. Thiringer has also demonstrated a close relationship between hypoxanthine concentrations in cerebral vein of the fetal sheep and the degree of asphyxia as indicated by increased lactate concentrations and deterioration of somatosensory evoked electroencephalogram potentials.

The findings of a close correlation between the degree of asphyxia and hypoxanthine concentrations have led to the suggestion that hypoxanthine might be a useful marker to assess the degree of asphyxia (Saugstad 1975).

ADENOSINE RELEASE IN THE NEWBORN INFANT

The adenosine concentration in the umbilical arterial blood in newborn infants was found to be 0.61 μmol/l $\pm$ 0.09 SEM (n=30), which is four-fold higher than in adults during resting condition (Irestedt, Sollevi & Lagercrantz, to be published). Even if this represents "normal" deliveries, we believe that the increased release of adenosine is due to the intermittent hypoxic periods during uterine contractions.

FUNCTIONAL EFFECTS OF AN ADENOSINE ANALOGUE

To study the functional effects of adenosine we have given an adenosine analogue: L-N^6-phenyl-isopropyladenosine (PIA) to rabbit pups and kittens and monitored their behaviour, respiration, temperature and oxygen consumption. This analogue is metabolically stable in contrast to adenosine which is very rapidly inactivated. Furthermore adenosine does not penetrate the blood-brain barrier as the analogue does. The adenosine analogue was given i.p. to the animals via an indwelling catheter. The animals were not anaesthetized and the ventilation was monitored by the barometric method, which is based on the recording of pressure changes in a closed box. The pressure changes are proportional to ventilation and caused by the heating of the inhaled air. To neutralize for environmental disturbances, the closed box was connected to a reference box of the same size (Drorbaugh & Fenn 1955).

We found that PIA caused a marked depression of respiration, particularly the respiratory rate; the effect on tidal volume was more variable. The effect of PIA was dose-dependent and lasted for more than 30 min. The youngest animals (1 and 3 days) seemed to be the most susceptible, while the effect was less marked in older animals (about 8 days) (see Fig. 1).

PIA also caused a drop of the body temperature (Fig. 2).

FIG. 1.

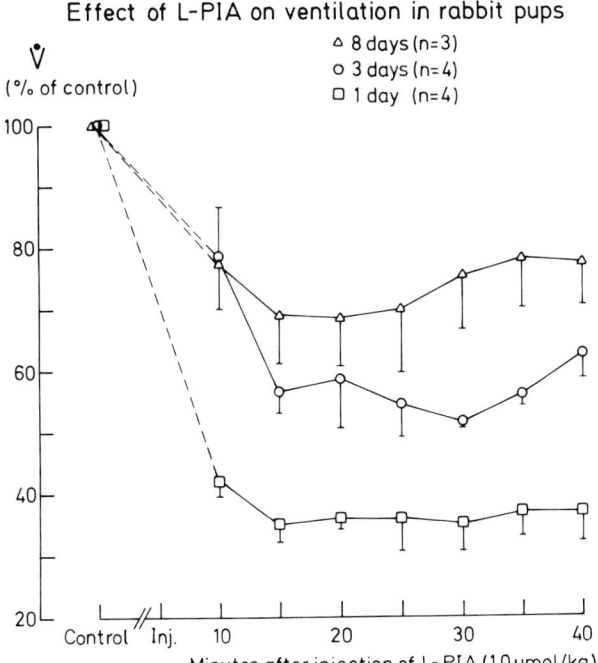

Ventilation ($\dot{V}$) monitored by the barometric method. The rabbit pups were non-anaesthetized and in sleep during the recording. The adenosine analogue (PIA) was given i.p. by an indwelling catheter. The bars represent one standard error of the mean (SEM). Chamber temperature: 28°C.

FIG. 2.

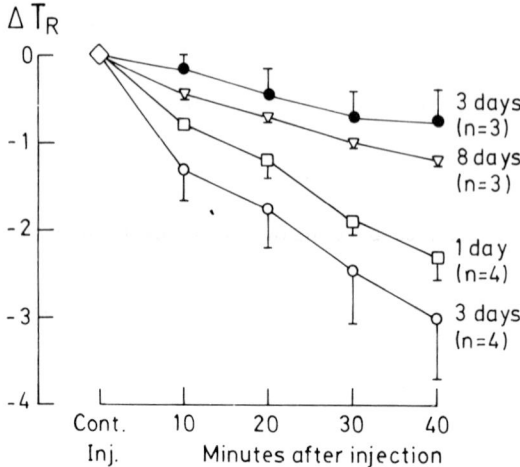

Change of rectal temperature ($T_R \pm$ SEM) after the administration of the adenosine analogue (PIA) i.p. by an indwelling catheter. Only a minor fall of the temperature was noted in three 3 day old pups pretreated with 10 mg/kg aminophylline (filled symbols).

This effect was marked when the animals were kept at around 28°C. When the chamber temperature was about 32°C the body temperature decreased only slightly. PIA also led to a decreased oxygen consumption (about 30 %) as measured with a modified Krogh spirometer.

The effect of PIA on respiration could thus partially be secondary to decreased metabolism. However, at a chamber temperature of 32°C there was a marked reduction of the ventilation in spite of a minute fall of body temperature indicating a direct respiratory effect of PIA. We also noted that the animals became drowsy and sedated after the injection of PIA.

All the above mentioned effect of PIA could be reversed after injection of aminophylline in a clinical dose (10 mg/kg body weight).

POSSIBLE FUNCTIONS OF ADENOSINE IN THE NEWBORN INFANT

It is tempting to speculate on the functional significance of endogenously released adenosine particularly during asphyxia.

The respiratory depression of asphyxiated newborn infants might be partially due to endogenously released adenosine. This well known hypoxic depression lasts longer than the period of asphyxia (Dawes 1968) and does not disappear directly after the arterial blood has been oxygenated, indicating that a chemical factor is acting in the brain-stem. Adenosine could be one such factor, although others e.g. endorphins and GABA might also be involved. However, the finding that the "hypoxic" depression can be antagonized with theophylline in the adult cat supports the idea that adenosine is the factor (Millhorn et al. 1984). The rapid decrease of temperature, hypotonia and sedation seen in newborn asphyxiated infants could also be partially due to adenosine. Adenosine can also contribute to the dilatation of the cerebral blood vessels and thus contribute to the brain swelling seen after asphyxia. Adenosine has indeed been shown to cause glial swelling (Bourke et al. 1983).

COUNTER-REGULATORY ROLE OF ADENOSINE VERSUS CATECHOLAMINES

During perinatal asphyxia remarkably high concentrations of catecholamines have been found both in fetal scalp blood samples and in umbilical arterial blood (Lagercrantz 1984). However, the effect of the high adrenaline concentrations on glycogenolysis and lipolysis seem to be considerably lower than in adults (Hägnevik et al. 1984). The blood pressure is, surprisingly, only slightly elevated in infants with high catecholamine levels (Faxelius et al. 1984). One possible explanation to these findings is that the released adenosine, which acts as an antilipolytic as well as a hypotensive agent, counteracts the effects of the catecholamines.

CONCLUSIONS

Adenosine is probably released during perinatal asphyxia in high concentrations, as indicated by the finding of high levels of the adenosine metabolite hypoxanthine after asphyxia. Adenosine has been shown to cause vasodilatation and hypotension, sedation, respiratory depression and hypothermia - all symptoms typical for perinatal asphyxia after birth. We have hypothetized that adenosine might be one chemical mediator of these symptoms. However, other neuroactive substances like the endorphins which also are released in higher concentrations during asphyxia might have similar effects and the relative importance of adenosine is probably variable due to species and gestational age.

ACKNOWLEDGEMENTS

Supported by the Swedish Medical Research Council (2553, 5234); Expressen's Prenatal Foundation and Sällskapet Barnavård.

RESUME

Au cours de l'asphyxie périnatale, et en particulier au moment de la naissance, apparaissent des neurohormones telles que, par exemple, les catécholamines, la vasopressine, et les endorphines, et sans doute aussi de fortes concentrations d'adénosine, substance qui pourrait être le médiateur des réactions à l'hypoxie (vasodilatation systémique, inhibition de la lipolyse et de la glycogénolyse, et dépression de la respiration.

L'adénosine est formée à partir des adénine-nucléotides dans de nombreux systèmes, dénotant une activité métabolique accrue, mais aussi au cours de l'hypoxie et en particulier dans le cerveau. Son métabolite, l'hypoxanthine, est retrouvé à des taux corrélés avec le degré d'asphyxie. Chez le nouveau-né, le taux d'adénosine dans le sang artériel ombilical est en moyenne de 0,61 μmol/l $\pm$0,09 SEM, après accouchement "normal"

L'étude des effets fonctionnels de l'adénosine a utilisé un analogue: la L-N^6-phényl-isopropyladénosine (PIA), administrée à des lapins et chats nouveau-nés par cathéter intravasculaire, sans anesthésie et avec enregistrement de la respiration. La PIA entraine une dépression respiratoire marquée, portant surtout sur la fréquence et moins sur le volume courant, dépression d'autant plus nette que l'animal est plus jeune; par ailleurs se produit une chute de la température rectale, surtout en milieu à 28°C, et une baisse de la consommation d'oxygène d'environ -30%. Tous ces effets sont abolis par une injection d'aminophylline à la dose de 10mg/kilo de poids.

La dépression respiratoire observée chez les enfants nés en état d'asphyxie pourrait être due en partie à la mise en circulation d'adénosine endogène. Cette hypothèse est renforcée par la notion de l'effet antagoniste de la théophylline chez le chat adulte soumis à une dépression respiratoire "hypoxique". L'adénosine pourrait aussi contribuer à la vasodilatation des vaisseaux cérébraux et favoriser ainsi l'oédème cérébral post-asphyxique.

Au cours de l'asphyxie périnatale, ont été relevés des taux sanguins remarquablement élevés de catécholamines, avec des effets lipolytiques et glycogénolytiques beaucoup plus faibles que chez l'adulte, et seulement une légère élévation de la pression artérielle: il est possible que ce soit l'adénosine mise en circulation qui contrecarre les effets des catécholamines.

Au total, l'adénosine peut être un des médiateurs chimiques du syndrôme post-asphyxique, mais d'autres substances neuroactives telles que les endorphines pourraient avoir des effets similaires; l'importance relative de l'adénosine varie probablement selon les espèces et l'âge gestationnel.

REFERENCES

Bourke, R.S., Kimelberg, H.K., Dazé, M. & Chuch, G. (1983): Swelling and ion uptake in cat cerebrocortical slices. Control by neurotransmitters and ion transport mechanisms. Neurochem.Res. 8, 5-24.
Burnstock, G. (1981): Purinergic receptors. Chapman & Hall, London.
Dawes, G. (1968): Fetal and neonatal physiology. Year Book Chicago.
Drorbaugh, J., & Fenn, W. (1955): A barometric method for measuring Ventilation in newborn infants. Pediatrics 16, 81-86.
Drury, A., & Szent-Györgyi, A. (1929): The physiological activity of adenine compounds with especial reference to their action upon the mammalian heart. J.Physiol.68, 213-237.
Eldridge, F., Millhorn, D., & Kiley, J. (1984): Respiratory effects of a long-acting analogue of adenosine. Brain.Res. 301, 273-280.
Faxelius, G., Lagercrantz, H., & Yao, A. (1984): Sympathoadrenal activity and peripheral blood flow after birth: comparison in infants delivered vaginally and by cesarean section. J.Pediatr.105, 144-148.
Fredholm, B.B. (1982): Adenosine receptors. Med.Biol.60, 289-293.
Hedner, T., Hedner, J., Wessberg, P., & Jonason, J. (1982) Regulation of breathing in the rat: indications for a role of central adenosine mechanisms. Neuroscience Letters 33, 147-151.
Hagnevik, K., Faxelius, G., Irestedt, H., Lagercrantz, H., Lundell, B., & Persson, B. (1984): Catecholamine surge and metabolic

adaptation in the newborn after vaginal delivery and caesarean section. Acta Paediatr.Scand. 73, 602-609.
Klein, R., Lagercrantz, H., & Zimmermann, H. eds (1982): Neurotransmitter Vesicles. Academic Press, London.
Lagercrantz, H. (1984): Catecholamine surge at birth in the human infant. In: Usdin, E., & Liss, A. eds, Proceedings of the 5th Catecholamine Symposium, New-York.
Lagercrantz, H., & Bistoletti, P. (1977): Catecholamine release in the newborn infant at birth. Pediatr.Res. 11, 889-893.
Lagercrantz, H., Yamamoto, Y., Fredholm, B.B., Prabhakar, N., & Euler, C.v. (1984): Adenosine analogues depress ventilation in rabbit neonates. Theophylline stimulation of respiration via adenosine receptors? Pediatr.Res.18, 387-390.
Millhorn, D., Eldridge, F., Kiley, J., & Waldrop, T. (1984): Prolonged inhibition of respiration following acute hypoxia in glomectomized cats. Resp.Physiol.57, 331-340.
Phillis, J., & Wu, P. (1981): The role of adenosine and its nucleotides in central synaptic transmission. Prog.Neurobiol. (Oxford) 16, 187-239.
Pohjavuori, M., & Fyhrquist, F. (1980): Hemodynamic significance of vasopressin in the newborn infant. J.Pediatr. 97, 462-465.
Saugstad, O. (1975): Hypoxanthine as a measurement of hypoxia. Pediatr.Res. 9, 158-161.
Thiringer, K. (1982): Hypoxanthine as a measure of fetal hypoxia. Academic thesis, Gothenburg.
Wardlaw, S., Stark, R., Baxi, L., & Frantz, A. (1979): Plasma beta-endorphin and beta-lipotropin in the human fetus at delivery: correlation with arterial pH and P_{O2}. J Clin.Endocrinol.Metab 49, 888-891.
Winn, R., Rubio, R., & Berne, R. (1981): Brain adenosine concentration during hypoxia in rats. Amer.J.Physiol.(Heart Circ. Physiol)241, H235-H242.

****

DISCUSSION. Dr.W.Oh, moderator.

Dr.Cl.Gautier: Did you look at the possible role of adenosine on the biphasic response to hypoxia in the neonatal period?

Dr.H.Lagercrantz: This is possible. But this response to mild hypoxia might not be due to adenosine because you cannot block it completely with theophylline. The adenosine response needs a substantial hypoxia such as in asphyxiated neonates with protracted apnea, or in preterm babies with repeated apneas who get hypoxic, then they might build up the adenosine concentration.

Dr.B.Lundell: You are using a rather high dose of theophylline. Is the effect of adenosine sustained after a single dose or do you have to amintain a certain plasma level?

Dr.H.Lagercrantz: We use 10 milligrams per kilogram of aminophylline, which is the same as used in clinical practice.

Dr.L.Stern: What do you propose as a mechanism for the theophylline action? Is there a competition for adenosine binding sites?

Dr.H.Lagercrantz: Yes, there is.

Dr.W.Oh: Which did you measure, A1 or A2?

Dr.H.Lagercrantz: A1 because we know that adenosine analogue acts mainly on the A1 receptors.

Dr.L.Stern: Is there any chemical similarity between adenosine and theophylline?

Dr.H.Lagercrantz: Yes, there is indeed some similarity.

Dr.P.Vert: First, can you exclude an indirect effect through an increase in blood flow? Second, do you know if adenosine is crossing the blood-brain brain barrier?

Dr.H.Lagercrantz: No, I cannot completely exclude that, but we have shown the same respiratory depressive effect of the adenosine analogue, after direct application in the fourth ventricle. Secondly adenosine does not cross the blood-brain barrier; however, the analogue PIA does!

Pr.P.Karlberg: Several years ago, Tim Oliver and I studied the neutral temperature for the neonate and recorded the oxygen consumption at different environmental temperatures (Amer.J.Dis.Child.1963; 105:427). We found in the normal ones an increased oxygen consumption at low temperature. But when we gave the newborn infant 16-17% oxygen to breathe, we did not record any metabolic response: they were dropping their body temperature. So that could be an effect of hypoxia. May the production of adenosine block the metabolic response?

Dr.H.Lagercrantz: It could be an explanation.

Factors influencing surfactant synthesis and release

Joseph B. Warshaw, Scott Jamison and Janice Sissom

The University of Texas Health Science Center at Dallas, 5323 Harry Hines Boulevard, Dallas, TX 75235, USA

ABSTRACT

Lung and placental maturation is delayed in offspring of diabetic rats. In lung of diabetic offspring a delay in glycogen depletion is associated with a lag in the maturation of surfactant synthesis. Placentas also show increased glycogen content and are 50% heavier than controls with an increase in DNA content. Both lung and placental membranes of diabetic offspring showed decreased EGF binding. Surfactant release from lung slices is stimulated by EGF in a calcium dependent mechanism. Other agents including prostaglandin E_2, isoproterenol and the phorbol ester TPA also stimulated release. Isoproterenol stimulated surfactant release from lung slices of 21 day fetuses of diabetics was less than in controls.

Our studies provide further evidence for a relationship between glycogen metabolism and surfactant phospholipid synthesis in the maturational delay seen in diabetic pregnancy. We also show that EGF has a regulatory influence on surfactant synthesis and secretion and has a likely role in placental growth.

KEYWORDS

Surfactant, lung development, diabetes, growth factors.

INTRODUCTION

Pulmonary surface active materials are essential for development and maintenance of alveolar stability in the immediate newborn period. Since the observations by Liggins (1969) that glucocorticosteroids stimulate lung maturation during development of the sheep fetus there have been numerous studies of influences of various hormones and growth factors on development of the surfactant system. Agents which have been reported to stimulate surfactant synthesis in vivo or in vitro include glucocorticosteroids (Rooney, Gobran, et al., 1979), thyroid hormones (Wu, et al., 1973), thyrotropin releasing hormones (Rooney, Marino, et al., 1979), estrogen (Khosla, et al., 1980), prolactin (Hamosh and Hamosh, 1977), β-adrenergic agents (Enhorning et al., 1977), cyclic AMP (Hallman, 1977), cholinergic agents (Brown and Longmore, 1981), prostaglandins (Marino and Rooney, 1980) and growth factors (Smith, 1979; Smith, et al., 1980, Sundell et al., 1975;

Catterton, et al., 1979). Most studies have been concerned with influences on the synthesis of surface active materials. Relatively little attention has been paid to factors associated with the release of the surfactant phospholipids by the type II cell.

While hyaline membrane disease is primarily a disorder of premature newborns, infants of diabetic mothers are particularly susceptible. The delay in lung maturation observed in infants of diabetic mothers prompted us to examine glycogen metabolism and phospholipid synthesis in offspring of streptozotocin induced diabetic rats. Robert et al. (1976) reported that human infants of diabetic mothers have a six-fold increase in the incidence of hyaline membrane disease as compared with normal controls until the 38th week of gestation.

In developing lung the glycogen content of lung falls prenatally coinciding with lung maturation and the late gestational surge in surfactant phospholipid synthesis. Bourbon and his colleagues (1982) have shown that glycogen is a substrate for surfactant synthesis during late fetal development. These relationships between glycogen depletion and phospholipid synthesis are delayed in fetuses of diabetic rats.

We have studied surfactant synthesis and release in normal animals and in a diabetic model in which lung maturation is delayed. These studies provide information concerning transmembrane signaling and further definition of the relationships between lung growth, substrate utilization, and phospholipid synthesis and release.

MATERIALS AND METHODS

Lung slices for studies of surfactant release are prepared from day 18-20 gestation fetal rats, using a McIlwain tissue chopper.

When type II cells were utilized, 1×10^6 cells are plated in 35 mm falcon dishes containing MEM and 10% fetal calf serum. The flasks are fitted with 0.5 mm inlets and outlets to permit subsequent perfusion of the cell in situ.

Perfusion of fetal lung

For studies of surfactant release, the lung slices (40-50 mg) are incubated for 1 hour at 37°C in 2 ml Krebs Ringer Phosphate containing 2 µCi ^{3}H-choline. At the end of this incubation period the lung slices are washed to remove excess ^{3}H-choline. The washed lung slices are then placed into the perfusion chambers made from 5 ml plastic syringes. 20-40 lung slices are distributed over a support grid (Ford mesh stainless steel) within the perfusion chamber. The chambers are then filled with 1.0 ml KRP. The chambers are sealed and perfused with 1 ml of aerated KRP/5 minutes using a multichannel peristalic pump until counts in the perfusate are stable. ^{3}H-Phosphatidylcholine content in the perfusate is determined after specific interventions. The system maintains pharmacological stability for 3-4 hours as determined by lactate dehydrogenase in the perfusate. Surfactant release can also be measured using cultured alveolar type II cells.

Lipid extraction from perfusate fractions was carried out by the method of Bligh and Dyer (1959). After drying, extracted lipids redissolved in chloroform are applied to thin layer plates as described previously and phosphatidylcholine determined after development of the chromatogram (Gilfillan, et al., 1983).

Preparation of streptozotocin diabetic rats

Females are made diabetic by intravenous injection of 40 mg/kg streptozotocin. Diabetic females are bred by placing them with stud males in cages overnight with mating confirmed by the presence of a copulatory plug and sperm. The morning after mating is arbitrarily designated as day 0 of gestation. Approximately 50% of attempted matings are successful.

Injection studies

For fetal injection studies pregnant control and diabetic rats are anesthetized with metofane and their uteri exposed by a small lateral suprpubic incision. EGF (100 ng) is injected directly into the amniotic sac through the uterine wall with a finely beveled Hamilton syringe. Only 3-4 fetuses on either side of the cervix are injected to minimize manipulation of the uterus. Separate pregnant animals are used for controls.

EGF binding

Membranes from lung and placenta were prepared by the method of Morishige et al. (1977).

For studies of EGF binding, lung and placental membranes (0.05 - 0.1 mg protein) are incubated with 0.4 ng ^{125}I-EGF containing 50,000 dpm in a binding buffer (Earles balanced salt solution, 15 mM Hepes, pH 7.8, 1% BSA) for 3 hours at 4°C. Nonspecific binding was determined by measuring counts bound after addition of an excess (1000 fold) of unlabelled EGF. Total assay volume is 0.25 ml. Competitive binding is determined by adding increasing amounts of unlabelled EGF. Excess ^{125}I-EGF is separated from bound EGF by centrifugation in a Beckman microfuge.

Glycogen content of tissues was determined by modification of the fluorometric method of Lowry and Passoneau (1972) as described previously (Maniscalco, et al., 1978). Protein was determined by the method of Lowry et al. (1951). EGF was obtained from Collaborative Research Co. (Cambridge, MA) and other reagents from commercial sources.

RESULTS

Maturational changes in diabetic offspring

Diabetic rats have a delay in the decrease of lung glycogen by 12 to 24 hours (Fig. 1). These changes have been related to a decrease in the active form of phosphorylase in the lung of diabetic offspring (Gewolb et al., 1982). Since fetal insulin levels in our studies did not differ significantly between diabetic and control offspring, fetal hyperglycemia per se appears to be the major factor responsible for delayed lung maturation. Fetal blood sugars of the diabetic animals were 355 mg% as compared with 51 mg% in controls (Gewolb et al., 1982). It is of interest that offspring of diabetics in this particular model had weights approximately 20% less than those of controls. All organs except the placenta were decreased in weight.

The placentas obtained from fetuses of streptozotocin diabetic rats showed marked alterations in glycogen content during the latter phases of the pregnancy. At term glycogen content of diabetic fetal placentas was higher than in control fetuses. Placental glycogen content was also related to changes in phosphorylase activity similar to what was observed in lung (Gewolb, et al., 1983). The weights of placentas from diabetic rats were approximately 50% heavier than controls. Also, placental DNA content continued to increase in the diabetic pregnancies until day 19 whereas DNA content was constant after day 16 in controls. It appears therefore that cell hyperplasia continues in the diabetic placenta, possibly under the influence of high glucose concentrations. The diabetic placentas not only contained more glycogen than controls but also exhibited histologic features normally seen earlier in gestation such as thickening of the trophoblastic layers. The thickening and modifications of the cellular barrier in the diabetic placentas may affect fetal growth and nutrition by increasing the diffusion distance between maternal and fetal circulations.

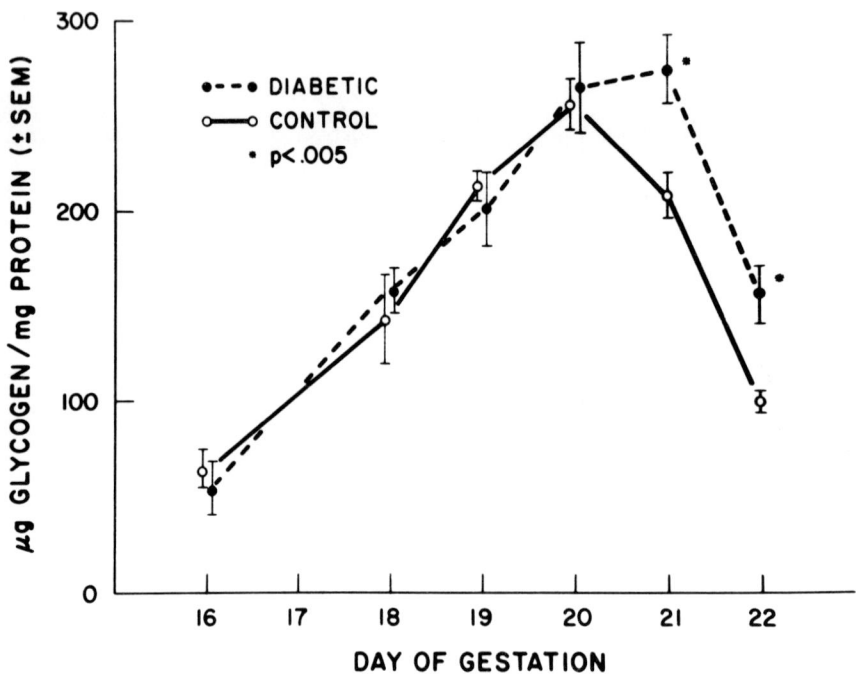

Fig. 1. Lung glycogen content in fetuses of diabetic and control pregnancies. From Gewolb et al., 1982.

Surfactant synthesis and release

Lung slices obtained from 21 day gestation of fetal rat lung were utilized for the superfusion experiments. Isoproterenol (10^{-4} to 10^{-6} M) caused a rapid and prompt increase in phosphatidylcholine release from both lung slices and isolated alveolar type II cells. A representative experiment is shown in Fig. 2. PGE_2 (10^{-6} M) caused a similar increase in phosphatidylcholine release. Prostaglandin E_2 stimulated release was completely inhibited by nifedipine (10^{-4} M), a potent calcium channel blocker. That surfactant release is controlled in major part by calcium fluxes is further supported by the observation that A 23187 (10^{-6} M), a calcium ionophore, also stimulated release of surfactant obtained from 21 day gestation fetal lung slices. Epidermal growth factor (10 ng/ml) stimulated surfactant release by lung slices and alveolar type II cells. Release stimulated by EGF was also calcium dependent. The phorbal ester, TPA (200 ng/ml), also stimulated surfactant release suggesting an effect mediated through protein kinase C.

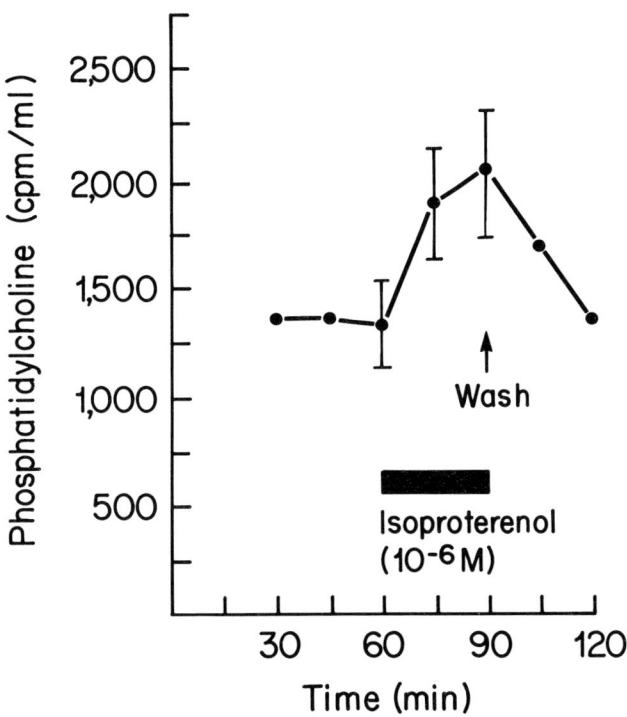

Fig. 2. Isoproterenol stimulated release of phosphotidylcholine from lung slices of 20 day gestation fetal rats. Slices are labelled with ^{3}H-choline, washed to remove excess ^{3}H-choline and exposed to isoproterenol as indicated.

We also investigated the release of phosphatidylcholine from lung slices obtained from 21 day gestation fetuses of diabetics. As shown in Fig. 3, consistent with previously reported data, incorporation of ^{3}H-choline into phospholipids isolated from lung of diabetic offspring was reduced. Isoproterenol stimulated surfactant release was greatly reduced in the diabetic as compared with release from normal controls.

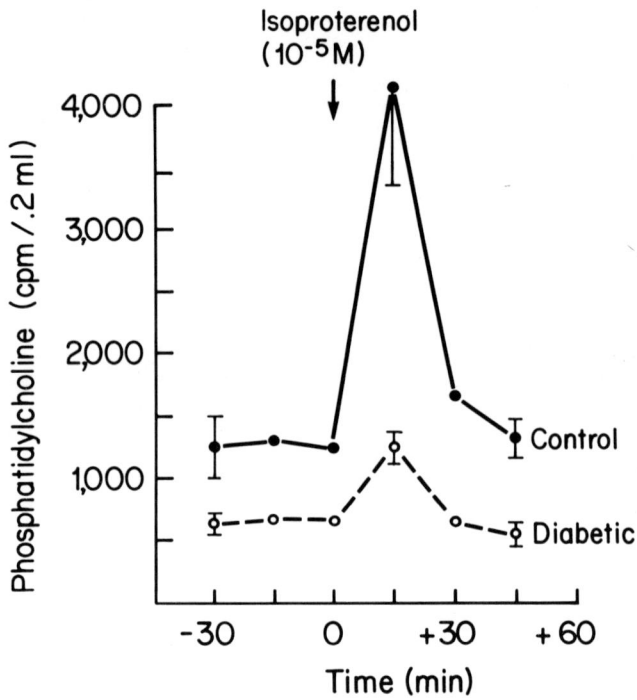

Fig. 3. Phosphatidylcholine release from lung slices prepared from 20 day gestation fetuses of diabetic and control rats. Conditions are those in Figure 2 and as described in the text.

Growth factor influences on surfactant release

Our own laboratory and others have demonstrated effects of epidermal growth factor on lung maturation (Sundell, et al., 1975, Warshaw, et al., 1985). EGF injected into the amniotic sac of 20 day gestation fetal rats results in a decrease in lung glycogen and enhancement of choline incorporation into phosphatidylcholine.

In addition to examining the effects of EGF on in vivo relationships between lung glycogen and phospholipid metabolism, we have also measured EGF binding to membrane fractions prepared from lung and placenta. EGF binds with high affinity to both lung and placenta. Our results indicate a reduction in EGF binding to membrane fractions isolated from placentas and lungs of fetuses of diabetic gestations.

DISCUSSION

The precise mechanism by which surfactant phospholipids packaged in lamellar bodies are secreted into the alveolus is unclear. Colcholine (Marino and Rooney, 1980) and vinblastin (Dobbs and Mason, 1978), agents which inhibit formation of microtubules also inhibit surfactant secretion. Also, Rooney's group (Marino and Rooney, 1980) has shown that the microfilament inhibitor, cytochalasin B, inhibits release of surfactant. These data suggest that these elements of the cytoskeleton are essential for surfactant release.

Our own studies and the results of others have demonstrated that diverse agents can stimulate surfactant release. While it is likely that the final pathways by which various hormones and factors affecting surfactant release involve exocytotic events associated with changes in the cytoskeleton, the precise intracellular mechanisms remain unknown.

These intracellular events may be mediated by calcium dependent enzymes. A central role for calcium is suggested by the observation that nifedipine, a calcium channel inhibitor, blocks prostaglandin and EGF stimulated increase in surfactant release from lung slices. Moreover, the calcium ionophore A23187 stimulated surfactant release directly.

We and others (Dobbs and Mason, 1978) have shown that phorbol esters stimulate surfactant release. These agents are analogues of naturally occurring diacylglycerol which modulates intracellular events by activating protein kinase C. Under the activity of specific lipases, phosphatidyinositol in the cell membrane generates diacylglycerol and inositol trisphosphate. The latter has a role in mobilizing intracellular calcium which may further amplify secretion of surfactant. The mechanism by which these compounds modulate surfactant release is uncertain.

EGF binds to specific receptors in developing lung (Adamson and Warshaw, 1982). Our data suggests a role for EGF in surfactant secretion as well as in enhancing late gestational lung maturation.

It is not clear at the present time whether the decrease in EGF binding to diabetic placenta and lung is directly related to the maturational delays exhibited in these tissues or is perhaps a direct effect of the hyperglycemic state in the developing diabetic fetus. We speculate that the decrease in placental EGF binding is related to the lack of maturation and the continued growth of the placenta in the diabetic condition of substrate excess. Since the large placenta may be ineffective in delivering substrates itself, there is growth retardation in the face of lung maturational delay. We have also found that while

EGF binding to placenta of diabetic offspring remains low throughout gestation, binding to lung increases to normal levels during the last 2-3 days of gestation (unpublished observation). Since these fetuses are mildly growth retarded possibly because of a relative decrease in nutrient transfer across the immature placenta in late gestation, enhancement of lung maturation at that time may be associated with an increase in EGF binding. This further supports the maturational role for EGF during late gestation.

REFERENCES

Adamson, E.G. and Warshaw, J.B. (1982): Down-regulation of epidermal growth factor receptors in mouse embryos. Dev. Biol. 90, 430-434.
Bligh, E.C. and Dyer, W.J. (1959): A rapid method of total lipid extraction and purification. Can. J. Biochem. Physiol. 37, 911-917.
Bourbon J.R., Rieutort, M., Engle, M.J. and Farrell, P.M. (1982): Utilization of glycogen for phospholipid synthesis in fetal rat lung. Biochim. Biophys. Acta 712, 382-389.
Brown, L.A.S. and Longmore, W.J. (1981): Adrenergic and cholinergic regulation of lung surfactant secretion in the isolated perfused rat lung and in the alveolar type II cell in culture. J. Biol. Chem. 256, 66-72.
Catterton, W.Z., Escobedo, M.B., Sexson, W.R., Gray, M.E., Sundell, H.W. and Stahlman, M.T. (1979): Effect of epidermal growth factor on lung maturation in fetal rabbits. Pediat. Res. 13, 104-108.
Dobbs, L.G. and Mason, R.J. (1978): Stimulation of secretion of disaturated phosphatidylcholine from isolated alveolar type II cells by 12-0-tetradecanoyl-13-phorbol acetate. Amer. Rev. Resp. Dis. 118, 705-713.
Enhorning, G., Chamberlain, D., Contreras, C., Burgoyne, R., and Robertson, B. (1977): Isoxsuprine-induced release of pulmonary surfactant in the rabbit fetus. Am. J. Obstet. Gynecol. 129, 197-202.
Gewolb, I.H., Barrett, C. and Warshaw, J.B. (1983): Placental growth and glycogen metabolism in streptozotocin diabetic rats. Pediat. Res. 17, 587-591.
Gewolb I.H., Barrett, C., Wilson, C.M. and Warshaw J.B. (1982): Delay in pulmonary glycogen degradation in fetuses of streptozotocin diabetic rats. Pediat. Res. 16, 869-873.
Gilfillan, A.M., Chu, A.J., Smart, D.A. and Rooney, S.A. (1983): Single plate separation of lung phospholipids including disaturated phosphatidylcholine. J. Lipid Res. 24, 1651-1655.
Hallman, M. (1977): Induction of of surfactant phosphatidylglycerol in the lung of fetal and newborn rabbits by dibutyryl adenosine 3':5'-monophosphate. Biochem. Biophys. Res. Commun. 77, 1094-1102.
Hamosh, M. and Hamosh, P. (1977): The effect of prolactin on the lecithin content of fetal rabbit lung. J. Clin. Invest. 59, 1002-1005.
Khosla, S.S., Gobran, L.I. and Rooney, S.A. (1980): Stimulation of phosphatidylcholine synthesis by 17β-estradiol in fetal rabbit lung. Biochim. Biophys. Acta 617, 282-290.
Liggins, G.C. (1969): Premature delivery of fetal lambs infused with glucocorticosteroids. J. Endocrin. 45, 515-523.
Lowry O.H. and Passoneau J.V. (1972): A flexible system of enzyme analysis. New York: Academic Press.
Lowry, O.H., Rosebrough, N.J., Farr, A.L. and Randall, R.J. (1951): Protein measurement with the folin phenol reagent. J. Biol. Chem. 193, 265-275 .
Maniscalco, W.M., Wilson, C.M., Gross, I., Gobran, L., Rooney, S.A., and Warshaw J.B. (1978): Development of glycogen and phospholipid metabolism in fetal and newborn rat lung. Biochim. Biophys. Acta 530, 333-346.
Marino, P.A. and Rooney, S.A. (1980): Surfactant secretion in a newborn rabbit lung slice model. Biochim. Biophys. Acta 620, 509-519.

Morishige, W.K., Uetake, C., Greenwood, F.C. and Akaka, J. (1977): Pulmonary insulin responsivity: in vivo effects of insulin on the diabetic rat lung and specific insulin binding to lung receptors in normal rats. Endocrinology 100, 1710-1722.

Robert, M.F., Neff, R.K., Hubbell, J.P., Taeusch, H.W. and Avery, M.E. (1976): Association between maternal diabetes and the respiratory-distress syndrome in the newborn. N. Engl. J. Med. 294, 357-360.

Rooney, S.A., Gobran, L.I., Marino, P.A., Maniscalco, W.M. and Gross, I. (1979): Effects of betamethasone on phospholipid content, composition and biosynthesis in fetal rabbit lung. Biochim. Biophys. Acta 572, 64-76.

Rooney, S.A., Marino, P.A., Gobran, L.I., Gross, I. and Warshaw, J.B. (1979): Thyrotropin-releasing hormone increases the amount of surfactant in lung lavage from fetal rabbits. Pediat. Res. 13, 623-625.

Smith, B.T. (1979): Lung maturation in the fetal rat: acceleration by injection of fibroblast-pneumocyte factor. Science 204, 1094-1095.

Smith B.T., Galaugher, W. and Thurlbeck, W.M. (1980): Serum from pneumnonectomized rabits stimulates alveolar type II cell proliferation in vitro. Am. Rev. Resp. Dis. 121, 701-707.

Sundell, H., Serenius, F., Barthe, T., Friedman, Z., Kanarek, K.S., Escobedo, M.B., Orth, D.N., and Stahlman, M.T. (1975): The effect of EGF on fetal lamb lung maturation. Pediat. Res. 9, 371.

Warshaw, J.B., Jamison, T.S., and Sissom J.F. (1985): EGF decreases lung glycogen and stimulates lung phosphatidylcholine synthesis in fetal rat. Pediat. Res., 19, 330.

Wu, B., Kikkawa Y., Orzalesi, M.M., Motoyama, E.K., Kaibara, M., Zigas, C.J. and Cook C.D. (1973): The effect of thyroxine on the maturation of fetal rabbit lungs. Biol. Neonate 22, 161-168.

RESUME

Les agents connus de stimulation de la synthèse du surfactant comprennent les glucocorticoides, les hormones thyroidiennes et la TRH, les oestrogènes, la prolactine, les beta-adrenergiques, l'AMP-cyclique, les cholinergiques, et les facteurs de croissance. Le retard de maturation pulmonaire noté chez les enfants de mère diabétique a conduit cette équipe à étudier le métabolisme du glycogène et la synthèse des phospholipides chez les produits de rates diabétiques (streptozocine).

La maturation pulmonaire et placentaire est retardée chez ces rats nouveau-nés. Dans le poumon, il existe un retard de 12-24 heures de la déplétion en glycogène, qui s'accompagne d'un décalage de la maturation de la synthèse du surfactant. L'hyperglycémie foetale (3,55 g/l contre 0,51 g/l chez les témoins) semble être la principale responsable de ce retard, les taux d'insuline foetale étant similaires. Les placentas des foetus de rates diabétiques ont un poids de 50% supérieur à celui des placentas témoins; leur contenu en glycogène est augmenté; leur contenu en DNA augmente jusqu'au 19e jour de gestation alors qu'il se stabilise à partir du 16e jour chez les témoins. Tant dans le poumon que dans les membranes placentaires, la liaison tissulaire de l'EGF ("epidermal growth factor") est diminuée. La libération du surfactant à partir des coupes de poumon est stimulée par l'EGF selon un mécanisme calcium-dépendant; elle est aussi déclenchée par la prostaglandine E2, l'isoprotérénol, et le TPA-ester de phorbol. Cependant, sous isoprotérénol, la libération de surfactant à partir du tissu pulmonaire, à 21 jours de gestation, est moindre chez les foetus de rate diabétique que chez les témoins.

Ces résultats comfirment la relation entre le métabolisme du glycogène et la synthèse des phospholipides du surfactant au cours du retard maturatif observé dans les grossesses de femmes diabétiques. Ils montrent aussi que l'EGF a une influence régulatrice sur la synthèse et la secrétion du surfactant, et qu'il joue probablement un rôle dans la croissance du placenta.

This work was supported by Research Grant 5 R01-HL-30119 from the National Heart, Lung, and Blood Institute of the National Institutes of Health.

****

DISCUSSION. Dr.W.Oh, moderator.

Pr.A.Minkowski: That was a fascinating paper involving maturation. I have two questions. First, last year at a seminar at the Pasteur Institute, EGF was largely discussed. Is EGF acting directly upon the calcium pool? Secondly, you showed data from infants of diabetic mothers. What happens in small-for-dates infants? Are the data reversed, or different? Is the mechanism modified?

Dr.J.Warshaw: Effects on calcium are likely not to be terribly specific to EGF. There are a number of ligand receptor interactions which are associated with changes in calcium flux. Calcium tends to be a common denominator for much of the signal transduction that takes place. The EGF effects which are likely to be more specific are those that relate directly to the effects of EGF on gene action after protein phosphorylation or receptor internalization. Newborn mice injected with EGF are smaller than controls.

Dr.J.Metcoff: That was a very interesting presentation. I have two questions. First, were the litter sizes the same in the diabetic and control mice?

Dr.J.Warshaw: The litter size in these animals is always very similar. We tried to control the litter effect.

Dr.J.Metcoff: Maybe it is a mistake to select comparison groups based on the litter size, because it selects the animals that you examine. In previous studies (J.Nutr.1981;$\underline{34}$:708), we found that in pregnant rats subjected to malnutrition, the litter size was significantly greater than that of the controls. Litters of the control rats were smaller and the pups were much larger. The total litter size and the total placental weights, however, were similar. The second question is: have you had any chance to measure DNA, protein, or RNA contents? Of course, the DNA content, particularly if you select the litter size, is directly proportional to placental weight.

Dr.J.Warshaw: Studies of surfactant release are <u>in vitro</u> experiments. We have also done work in which EGF is injected into the amniotic sac and in a second procedure ^{3}H-thymidine is injected into the animals. Preliminary experiments suggest that there is less DNA synthesis after EGF injection but we have much more work to do here.

Dr.W.Oh: What is the role of hormones in relation to EGF, cortisol for example?

Dr.J.Warshaw: Cortisol seems to increase the number of EGF receptors. However, the control of release is not as simple as that. The lung responds to a variety of input signals. The mechanisms involved in regulation of synthesis and release are not going to depend upon only one agent. Calcium again seems to be the important modulator.

Pr.P.Karlberg: What is causing the changed growth rate at 16 days?

Dr.J.Warshaw: My original speculation was that these effects on growth were due to high glucose levels. In association with this, we find a decrease in EGF binding. If EGF has a maturational influence, we may simply be seeing growth rather than maturation. There are also other growth factors which interact with these EGF receptors which are made by the placenta. These interactions may influence binding of EGF itself and growth.

Dr.L.Stern: You showed that interesting relationship between maturation and arrest of replication of DNA.

Dr.J.Warshaw: There is a general view that maturation occurs as growth decreases. Studies of cortisol influences on lung maturation show that with stimulation of maturation the DNA content of lung decreases.

Dr.L.Stern: All effective agents, e.g. cortisol, thyroxin, as well as heroin, inhibit lung growth.

Dr.W.Oh: Your model, hyperglycemia without hyperinsulinemia, is really a unique one. With a real model of hyperglycemia and hyperinsulinemia, what would you expect the EGF would do?

Dr.J.Warshaw: I think it would do the same thing. High insulin levels certainly increase the substrate flux. In that instance, it may be the substrate uptake that is most important and not insulin. In our studies, the fetuses are in fact growth-retarded but with very large placentas. The immature large placentas may restrict thet substrate delivery to the fetus.

Dr.J.P.Relier: Mikko Hallman heavily insists on the role of myoinositol as a growing factor for the lung; in his experiments, he gave a myoinositol-free diet to pregnant rabbits and some does had growth-retarded litters with stiking lung hypoplasia (in"Respiratory Distress Syndrome",Raivio Hallman Kouvalainen Valimaki Eds,Academic Press 1984, pp.33-50). Have you noticed any relationship between EGF and myoinositol?

Dr.J.Warshaw: We have not looked at that yet. We plan to examine phosphatidylinositol turnover.

Dr.J.P.Relier: This is an important practical and clinical point: Do you think we might, at the present time, give myoinositol in parenteral nutrition? It seems that there is no myoinositol in the industrial milk.

Dr.J.Warshaw: I would put inositol in the same category as carnitine and taurine, not of likely importance in milk.

Dr.J.Bourbon: Do you think that the main role of EGF is on surfactant secretion or synthesis?

Dr.J.Warshaw: I think it has an effect on both. The injection studies show that EGF has an effect on syhthesis. The effect on secretion is less specific with the common denominator being calcium.

Dr.J.Bourbon: It seems to exist a redundancy of systems for the surfactant secretion. How do you conceive that physiological process? And what could be the physiological role of EGF in this system?

Dr.J.Warshaw: EGF may be important for the entire maturational process. There are, however, likely to be many signals.

Dr.J.Bourbon: Your results and also the work we did with Philip Farrell (Biochem.Biophys.Acta 1982 712:382) suggest that glycogen is a preferential substrate for surfactant elaboration. How could you explain that glycogen is preferentially used rather than glucose, for example?

Dr.J.Warshaw: This is not just for surfactant. Glycogen is likely important for the other morphogenic events in lung.

Differentiation of type II pneumonocytes in immature rat lung studied by means of intra-embryonic grafting and *in vitro* culture

L. Marin, F. Dameron, M.E. Dufour and N. Guettari

INSERM U 29, Hôpital Port-Royal, 75674 Paris Cedex 14, France

ABSTRACT

For the past decade, it has been widely admitted that the differentiation of type II pneumonocytes within the respiratory epithelium depends on hormonal factors. Yet, recent experiments suggest that these factors do not trigger type II cell differentiation. We reinvestigated this problem first by grafting immature fetal rat lungs into developing embryos, then by explanting them *in vitro*. The developmental levels achieved in these conditions were assessed by means of electron microscopy. The results showed that type II cells, containing specific lamellar inclusion bodies differentiated in grafted lungs, as well as *in vitro*. When compared to normal *in vivo* development, the timing of differentiation was delayed in grafted lungs, whereas it was accelerated *in vitro*. These results support the hypothesis that hormonal factors are not involved in the process initiating type II cell differentiation. They also suggest that inhibitory factors participate in the control of differentiation timing *in vivo*.

KEY-WORDS

Lung development, type II cells, rat fetus.

INTRODUCTION

The differentiation of type II pneumonocytes in the course of fetal lung development is the morphological expression of the onset of surfactant synthesis (Askin and Kuhn, 1971; Balis and Conen, 1964) representing a major event in the processes of functional lung maturation. The aim of most experimental studies in this field during the past few years has therefore been to acquire a better knowledge of these cells, especially about the factors triggering and regulating their appearance and differentiation.

Fetal lung maturation was first stimulated by Liggins (1968) who infused corticosteroids into lambs maintained *in utero*. Since then, a considerable amount of developmental studies has led to the idea, now widely accepted, that maturational processes, particularly type

II cell differentiation, depend greatly on hormonal factors. Corticosteroids were first and extensively investigated but it gradually appeared that a number of other hormones might equally be involved in the control of lung maturation (for a review, see Gross, 1984; Hitchcock, 1980; Smith, 1984). Despite the tremendous efforts that have been undertaken to elucidate the mechanisms underlying the endocrine control of lung maturation, many aspects of these problems remain unclear. Whereas the regulatory function of hormones has indeed been proved once distal epithelial cells have started to differentiate into type II pneumonocytes, one still knows very little about the factors triggering the appearance of these cells. We reinvestigated this problem using an _in vivo_ culture system, the intra-embryonic graft method (Marin et al., 1981) which offers a number of advantages: the transplanted fetal tissues continue to develop under close-to-natural conditions since they are kept in a living and fetal environment throughout the experiment; the relationships between the various cell types are maintained; finally, the grafted tissue is rapidly colonized by the recipient's circulation. Therefore, all systemic factors provided by the host, whether they are stimulating or inhibiting factors, reach the differentiating cells of the grafted tissue through the normal way, i.e. via the blood stream.

In the work reported in this paper, we compared the results obtained with this method with those gained from _in vitro_ experiments. The developmental level achieved by immature rat lung tissue, when grafted or cultured, was assessed by an electron microscopic study.

METHODS

Animals
Sprague-Dawley female rats were mated overnight; the next morning was considered day 0 of gestation. Fetuses were delivered by cesarean section on days 13, 16, 17, and 18 of gestation. They were killed by decapitation; their lungs were dissected and kept in saline until grafting or culture.

Grafting
Only the middle lobe of the right lung was used. The tissue was cut into pieces of 0.5 mm3; For each fetus, 3 samples taken at random were kept for grafting into chick embryos. These embryos had been incubated for $3\frac{1}{2}$ days. At that stage, their vascular network was sufficiently developed to enable a rapid colonization of the graft. On the other hand, possible circulating hormones were still at a very low level (Kalliecharan and Hall, 1974). An incision was made in the side of the embryo, and a piece of fetal rat lung was inserted into it. The eggs containing the graft-bearing embryos were further incubated for given periods of time. The grafted lungs were recovered when they were theoretically aged 19, 20, and 21 days of total gestation. Therefore, the grafting duration was the difference between gestational age at the explant time and total gestation.

Culture
Lungs from 13 or 16 day old rat fetuses were dissected, then cut into 0.5 mm3 cubes using a Mc Ilwain tissue chopper. They were then distributed on a gelified culture medium, Waymonth's alone or Waymonth's supplemented with 10% fetal calf serum. Penicillin (100 u/ml) and streptomycin (0.1 mg/ml) were added to both culture media. Explants were recovered when they were equivalent to 17 or

19 days of gestation.

Electron microscopy
Recovered lung grafts or explants were rapidly cut into 2 to 4 pieces, according to their size. They were fixed by immersion in ice-cold Hirsch and Fedorko's fixative (1968), dehydrated in graded acetone and embedded in Epon. Semi-thin sections were prepared from all blocks, stained with toluidine blue and examined by light microscopy. Thin sections were prepared using a LKB ultramicrotome, stained with uranyl acetate and lead citrate, and examined with a Hitachi HS 9 electron microscope.

RESULTS

I. Grafted lungs
In the experiments reported in this paper, the graft-bearing chick embryos were no older than $8\frac{1}{2}$ days of incubation at the time of their sacrifice. In most cases the grafted lung tissue was easily recognized from the chick tissue. Due to the relatively short grafting period (5 days or less), up to 60-70% of the initial transplants were recovered. Usually these appeared as round translucent masses, white or faintly pinkish, and they contained a clearly discernible epithelial network and a more or less developed vascular system. The actual growth of the transplants was not measured. Because these specimens had to be cut into pieces of about the same volume as the initial grafts, for electron microscopy, the volume increase could be estimated. This increase was maximum (about 4 times) when fetal rat lung tissue was transplanted at an early stage (16 days of gestation). When transplanted tissue was taken from 17 or 18 day old rat fetuses, the transplant volume increase was never more than 2-fold.

The developmental level was first assessed by examining semi-thin sections from all blocks. At the time of grafting, transplanted lung tissue was completely immature. In particular, no epithelial cell had differentiated into type II pneumonocytes, as these cells first appear on day 19 (Williams, 1977).

When they were recovered, mesodermal cells had accumulated lipid vacuoles, as can be seen in the course of normal development (Marin et al., 1982; Tordet et al., 1981; Vaccaro and Brody, 1978). As to the epithelium, the developmental stage achieved during grafting depended on the original stage of the transplants, and on the duration of grafting. When transplants were recovered at a stage equivalent to 19 days of gestation, the well developed epithelial network was still pseudoglandular, whatever the original stage of the grafted tissue. When transplants were recovered at a stage equivalent to 20 days of gestation, in those which originated from 16 day old fetuses, the epithelium was still high, whereas in transplanted tissue taken from 17 and 18 day old fetuses, the epithelium had flattened and looked intermediate between the pseudoglandular and the canalicular stages of normal development. In all three series, some epithelial cells contained dark inclusions representing lamellar bodies specific for differentiated type II pneumonocytes. In transplants recovered at a stage equivalent to 21 days of gestation, the number of inclusion-containing cells had increased in all series. But the proportion of epithelial cells which had transformed into type II pneumonocytes depended on the original stage of the transplants (Table I).

Table I. Percentage of inclusion containing epithelial cells in transplanted lung primordia fixed when they were theoretically 21 days old.

Original stage of transplanted lungs (days of gestation)	16 days	17 days	18 days
Duration of grafting	5 days	4 days	3 days
Number of recovered transplants	16	12	12
Total number of epithelial cells examined	2545	1302	1164
Total number of inclusion containing epithelial cells	295	164	273
Percentage	11.6%	12.6%	23.5%

The older the lung tissue was at transplantation time, the higher was the percentage of type II cells.

The electron microscopic control of these experiments confirmed the histological observations. All cells, whether they had differentiated or not, looked normal. In particular, mesodermal interstitial cells were loaded with lipidic vacuoles (Fig.1), as they normally are during the perinatal period in the rat. Like in normal lung, these lipid containing fibroblasts were lying between the vascular endothelium and the epithelium (Marin et al., 1982).

Epithelial cells were usually loaded with glycogen; their Golgi system and RER were well developed; intercellular junction types appeared to be like those in normal lung. In addition, in a number of transplants, perfectly normal type II cells, containing osmiophilic lamellar bodies, were found. As seen in figure 1, these type II pneumonocytes closely resembled those found in normal fetal rat lung. The osmiophilic lamellar bodies (Fig.2) were structurally identical to the inclusions appearing in the course of normal development. Moreover, in some transplants, they were released in the lumina where they transformed into typical "tubular myelin" (Fig.3).

Therefore, although the grafted fetal lung tissue remained in a medium containing at best highly diluted hormones, the differentiation of perfectly normal type II cells did take place.

II. <u>In vitro culture</u>

In a first series of experiments, lung tissue from 16 day old fetuses was grown in a chemically defined medium, without addition of serum or hormones. In this series, explants were cultured for 3 days, i.e. until a stage equivalent to 19 days of gestation. As recently reported by Gross and Wilson (1983), these explants did differentiate. In particular, a number of epithelial cells had

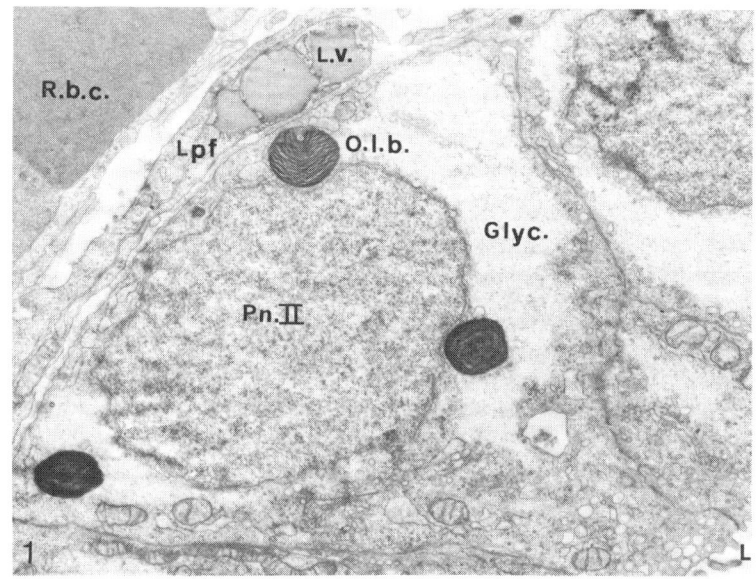

```
Glyc: glycogen
L   : lumen
Lpf :lipofibro-
        blast
L.v.: lipidic
        vacuole
O.l.b.:osmiophilic
        lamellar
        body
Pn.II:type II
        pneumonocyte
R.b.c;red blood
        cell
```

Figure 1. Rat lung tissue explanted from a 16 day old rat fetus and grafted for 4 days. Some epithelial cells have differentiated into normal type II pneumonocytes. Mesoderm cells lyong between them and the vascular wall have accumulated lipid vacuoles. x 8 000.

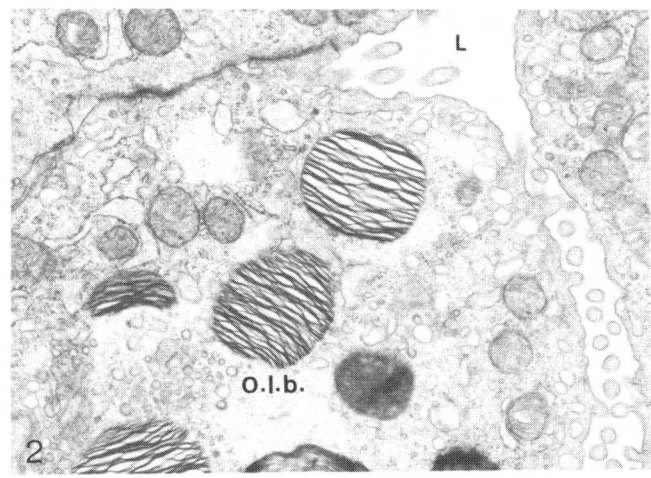

```
L  : lumen
O;l.b. : osmiophilic
        lamellar body
```

Figure 2. Rat lung tissue explanted from a 18 day old rat fetus and grafted for 3 days. Typical lamellar bodies have differentiated within epithelial cells. x 16 000.

transformed into type II cells (Fig.4). In addition, when compared with <u>in vivo</u> development, these type II cells looked "overdifferentiated", suggesting either an amplification or an anticipation of the differentiation processes.

In order to elucidate this last point, in a second set of experiments we explanted lung primordia of 13 day old rat fetuses, and recovered

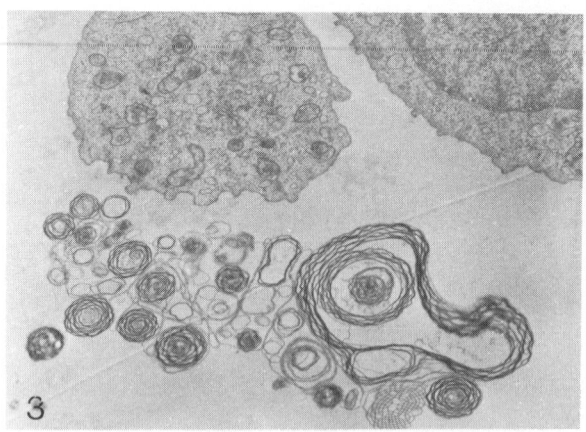

Figure 3. Rat lung tissue explanted from a 8 day old fetus and grafted for 3 days. Lamellar bodies have been released in the lumen. x 8 000.

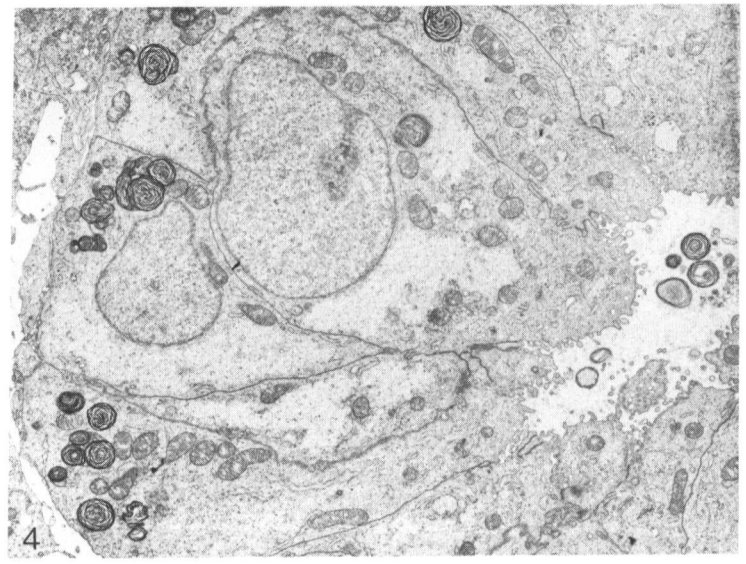

Figure 4. Rat lung tissue from a 16 day old fetus explanted for 3 d days, on Waymonth's medium. Epithelial cells contain numerous osmiophilic lamellar bodies. x 7 000.

them at a stage equivalent to 17 days of gestation, i.e. 48 hours before the normal appearance of type II cells. In this series, fetal calf serum was usually added to the culture medium to ensure a better survival of tissues. As seen in figure 5, type II cells containing osmiophilic lamellar bodies had différentiated. When lung primordia were grown without serum, the same result was obtained as long as they survived.

Thus, not only can undifferentiated epithelium transform into type II cells in vitro, but when compared to normal in vivo development, this

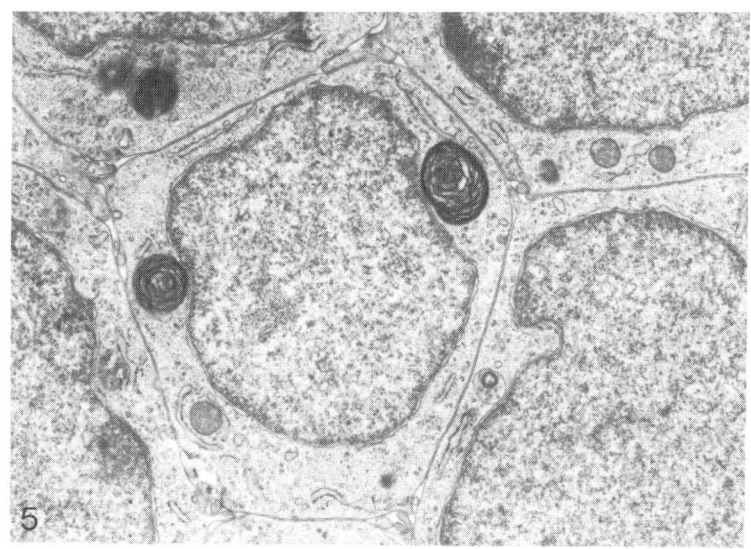

Figure 5. Rat lung tissue from a 13 day old rat fetus explanted for 4 days (i.e. equivalent to 17 days of gestation old). Epithelial cells were transforming into type II pneumonocytes.   x 10 000.

evolution is accelerated.

DISCUSSION

As shown by the reported data, completely immature fetal rat lung tissue is able to differentiate when withdrawn from its original organism, a result which could be expected from a number of previous in vitro experiments. The additional use of the intra-embryonic grafting has demonstrated that the timing and level of this differentiation depend on the initial stage of the grafted lung tissue.

Very little is known about the possible hormones or other circulating factors which might be found in the chick embryos at the early stages used in our experiments. Indeed, at least two hormones of maternal origin have been found in non-incubated eggs: an insulin-like factor (Trenkle and Hopkins, 1971), localized in the albumen, and thyroxin, stored in the yolk (Hilfer and Searls, 1980). But as far as we know, the actual levels of circulating hormones thought to be involved in the control of lung maturation have not been measured at the very young stages of chick development. Circulating corticosteroids on the one hand (Kalliecharan and Hall, 1974), plasma thyroxin on the other hand (Gaspard et al., 1981; Hilfer and Searls, 1980; Thommes et al., 1977) have been measured starting only on day 9 of incubation. At this time, the measured levels are very low when compared either to those measured in older chick embryos (Hilfer and Searls, 1980; Kalliecharan and Hall, 1974; Thommes et al.,1977), or to those in the fetal rats (Cohen,1973; Fisher et al.,1977). Therefore, in our graft bearing embryos, which were never older than $8\frac{1}{2}$ days of incubation, the levels of circulating hormones are, at maximum, equal to those measured on day 9. In fact, these levels most probably are lower. Hence the immature rat lung primordia which have been transplanted into chick embryos have differentiated in an environment which contained, at best, highly diluted hormones.

As already said, the type II pneumonocytes which appeared in these conditions closely resembled those appearing during normal development. Spatial relationships with other lung cells were maintained throughout the experiment. Despite this fact, the timing of the differentiation was slowed down when compared to normal development: OLBs which normally appear on day 19 of gestation were never found in transplants whose stage was equivalent to 19 days. They first appeared on day 20, and only in a few epithelial cells. This delay might of course result from the manipulations involved in the transplantation procedures; it also might be due to the fact that the fetal environment found in a chick embryo is but grossly equivalent to that in the fetal rat. But it must be pointed out that, when fetal lung tissue is grown in vitro, the transplantation procedures are, at least , as harmful as for in vivo experiments. Furthermore the in vitro environment is in many respects even more different from the in vivo conditions. Yet, as shown by previous reports involving human fetal lung (Mendelson et al., 1981), and by the above reported results, the differentiation timing is accelerated in vitro.

In conclusion, these results support the hypothesis that factors other than the fetal endocrine system are involved in the initiation of type II cell differentiation. The fact that lung maturation is delayed when lung tissue is grafted within a young growing embryo, whereas it is accelerated in vitro, suggests that in vivo some inhibitory factors are involved in the control of early lung development, thus contributing in the regulation of the timing of lung cells differentiation.

RESUME

On admet très généralement de puis une dizaine d'années que la maturation de l'épithélium respiratoire pendant la vie foetale, en particulier celle des pneumocytes de type II, se trouve sous le contrôle de facteurs hormonaux. S'il est vrai que diverses hormones exogènes stimulent la maturation lorsque celle-ci est amorcée, l'intervention de ces facteurs dans le contrôle de l'initiation de la différentiation ne semble pas démontrée. Nous avons repris ce problème soit en greffant du tissu pulmonaire indifférencié dans de jeunes embryons de poulet, soit en explantant ce tissu in vitro. Le tissu greffé a été prélevé sur des foetus de rat de 16, 17, et 18 jpurs de gestation, et maintenu en greffe jusqu'à ce qu'il ait atteint un stade équivalent à 19, 20 et 21 jpurs de gestation (c.à.d. jusqu'au moment où les pneumocytes de type II apparaissent et se différencient). Le tissu pulmonaire explanté in vitro a été prélevé sur des foetus de rat de 16 ou 13 jours de gestation, et maintenu en culture jusqu'à un stade équivalent à 19 ou à 16 jours de gestation. L'examen en microscopie électronique des greffons ou des explants recueillis a montré que: 1) En greffe, le tissu pulmonaire immature s'est différencié, bien qu'il ait été maintenu dans un milieu pratiquement anhormonal pendant toute la durée de l'expérience. Toutefois cette différentiation s'est déroulée avec retard par rapport rapport au développement normal, et ceci d'autant plus que le tissu greffé avait été prélevé sur un foetus plus jeune. 2) En culture, l'épithélium s'est également différencié, que le milieu contienne ou non du sérum. En outre, cette différenciation s'est déroulée plus rapidement qu'_in vivo_. L'ensemble de ces résultats suggère que les facteurs endocriniens ne sont pas impliqués dans les processus d'initiation de la différenciation des pneumocytes de type II. Ces résultats suggèrent aussi que des facteurs de type inhibiteur participent au contrôle de la chronologie de la différentiation au cours du développement foetal normal.

ACKNOWLEDGMENT

We are grateful to Dr.Diane Andrews (New-York) for reviewing the manuscript.

REFERENCES

Askin, F.B.,Kuhn, C.(1971): The cellular origin of pulmonary surfactant. Lab.Invest. 25, 260-269.
Balis, J., Conen, P.E.(1964): The role of alveolar inclusion bodies in the developing lung. Lab.Invest.13, 1215-1229.
Cohen, A.(1973): Plasma corticosterone concentration in the fetal rat. Horm.Metab.Res.5, 66-70
Fisher, D.A., Dussault, J.H., Sack, J., et al.(1977): Ontogenesis of hypothalamic-pituitary-thyroid function and metabolism in man, sheep and rat. Rec.Prog.Horm.Res.33, 59-116.
Funckhouser, J.D., Hughes, E.R.(1978): Differentiation of the pulmonary surfactant system. Disaturated phosphatidylcholine accumulation in fetal rat lung _in vivo_ and _in vitro_. Biochem. Biophys.Acta 530, 9-16.
Gaspard, K.J., Klitgaard, H.M., Wondergem, R.(1981): Somatomedin and thyroid hormones in the developing chick embryo. Proc.Soc.Exp.Biol. Med.166, 24-27.
Gross, I.(1984): Regulation of fetal lung maturation: initiation and modulation. In Respiratory Distress Syndrome, Raivio, Hallman, Kouvalainen and Välimäki ed., pp 51-64. Academic Press.
Gross, I., Wilson, C.(1983): Fetal rat lung maturation: initiation and modulation. J.Appl.Physiol.Respirat.Environ.55, 1725-1732.
Hilfer, S.R., Searls R.L.(1980): Differentiation of the thyroid in the hypophysectomized chick embryo. Develop.Biol.79, 107-118.
Hirsch, J.G., Fedorko, M.E.(1968): Ultrastructure of human leucocytes after simultaneous fixation with glutaraldehyde and osmium tetroxyde and post-fixation in uranyl-acetate. J.Cell.Biol.38, 625-627.
Hitchcock, K.R.(1980): Lung development and the pulmonary surfactant system: hormonal influences. Anat.Rec.198, 13-34.
Kalliecharan, R., Hall, B.K.(1974): A developmental study of the levels of progesterone, corticosterone, cortisol and cortisone circulating in plasma of chick embryos. Gen.Comp.Endocrinol.24, 364-372.
Liggins G.C.(1968): Premature parturition after infusion of corticotropin or cortisol into fetal lambs. J.Endocrinol.42, 323-329.
Marin, L., Dameron, F.L., Relier, J.P.(1981): Le surfactant pulmonaire au cours du développement foetal et néonatal. Rôle des facteurs humoraux foetaux. In Biologie du Développement, A.Minkowski Ed., pp 27-57. Paris: Flammarion.
Marin, L., Dameron F.L., Relier J.P.(1982): Changes in the cellular environment of differentiating type II pneumocytes. A quantitative study in the perinatal rat lung. Biol.Neonate 41, 171-182.

Mendelson, C.R., Johnston, J.M., McDonald, P., Snyder J.M.(1981):
   Multihormonal regulation of surfactant synthesis by human fetal
   lung in vitro. J.Clin.Endocrinol.Metabol.53, 307-317.
Minor, R.R.(1979): Organ cultures of embryonic lung tissues.
   J.Peditr.95, 910-916.
Smith, B.T.(1984): Pulmonary surfactant during fetal development and
   neonatal adaptation: hormonal control. In Pulmonary Surfactant,
   Robertson, VanGolde, Batenburg Ed., pp 357-381. Amsterdam: Elsevier
Snyder, J.M., Mendelson, C.R., Johnston, J.M.(1981): The effect of
   cortisol on rabbit fetal lung maturation in vitro. Develop.Biol.
   85, 129-140.
Thommes, R.C., Vieth R.L., Levasseur, S.(1977): The effects of
   hypophysectomy by means of surgical decapitation on thyroid
   function in the developing chick embryo. I. Plasma thyroxin. Gen.
   Comp.Endocrinol.31, 29-36.
Tordet, C., Marin, L., Dameron, F.L.(1981): Pulmonary di- and tri-
   acylglycerols during the perinatal development of the rat.
   Experientia 37, 333-334.
Trenkle, A., Hopkins K.(1971): Immunological investigation of an
   insulin-like substance in the chicken egg. Gen.Comp.Endocrinol.16,,
   493-497.
Vaccaro, C., Brody, J.S.(1978): Ultrastructure of developing alveoli.
   I. The role of the interstitial fibroblast. Anat.Rec.192, 467-481.
Williams, M.C.(1977): Development of the alveolar structure of the
   fetal rat in late gestation. Fed.Proc.36, 2653-2659.

****

DISCUSSION. Dr.W.Oh, moderator.

Dr.J.Warshaw: These results are very similar to data from Snyder et
al.(Cell Tissue Res 1981; 220:17); they utilized lungs from first
trimester human fetuses. After 7 days in explant culture, these lungs
went through the same kind of maturational advances, maybe because of
the absence of inhibitory hormones. So circulating hormones are not
necessary for maturation. The lung itself may make maturational
factors, EGF for example.

Mme L.Marin: The interesting point is that when a tissue is grafted
into a chicken embryo, maturation is delayed; the more undifferentiated the grafted lung, the longer the delay will be.

Dr.J.Warshaw: Have you tried to grow explants in the presence of
chick embryo extracts to see whether there is anything in the chicken
that does this?

Mme L.Marin: No, but we could do it, of course.

Perinatal pharmacology
Pharmacologie périnatale

John Lind and perinatal pharmacology

L.O. Boréus

Departments of Pediatrics and Clinical Pharmacology, Karolinska Hospital, Stockholm S-10401, Sweden

ABSTRACT

Since the 1950's new pharmacotherapeutic possibilities appeared in "adult" medicine, but they had to translated in terms of pediatric pharmacologic data. The main achievement has been quantitation with sensitive, selective, and reliable technics. The role of pharmaceutical formulation has been pointed out. The knowledge of drug metabolism into active metabolites has important implications for both fetal and neonatal pharmacology (e.g. theophylline). Species differences may be so large that animal studies bear little significance to human perinatology. Inter-individual variations are large and alternative routes for biotransformation allow flexibility. More controlled clinical trials in children are needed and they can be designed with the minimal risk and discomfort, especially with the help of noninvasive methods.

KEY-WORDS
Pediatric pharmacology, drug metabolism, fetus, neonate, theophylline, species differences, ductus arteriosus, catecholamines, ligand binding, phenobarbital.

INTRODUCTION

John Lind was a man with visions. He always seemed to anticipate the future directions and areas in pediatric research. He had an intuitive feeling about what was waiting around the corner.

One day, now 24 years ago, I went up to Johnny and asked him if he would be interested in setting up a unit for Clinical Pharmacology in his Pediatric Department at the Karolinska Hospital. He immediately responded with enthusiasm and set aside a laboratory and an office in his already somewhat overcrowded clinic. We called this unit the Clinical Pharmacology Lab. This was the beginning of a stimulating and joyful cooperation with Johnny which lasted for more than two decades. The best way for me to honour Johnny at this Symposium might be to point out some major things that have happened in clinical pediatric pharmacology during these 20 years. Johnny was a devoted internationalist and my review will therefore be made from an international perspective.

HISTORY

At the end of the 1950's, drug therapy in pediatrics was still mainly empirical and based on inherited clinical experience. But things were bound to change when new pharmacotherapeutic possibilities appeared in "adult" medicine. These possibilities had to be exploited also in pediatrics but the dictionary for translation of pharmacologic data from adults to children, especially newborn infants, was not at hand. This was demonstrated on a large scale by the chloramphenicol disaster.

At the beginning of the 1960's, there was little activity within pediatric pharmacology in Europe. In the United States there seemed to be a growing understanding that the issue was important. Harry Shirkey's "Pediatric Therapy" had appeared in its first edition in 1964. It was apparent that a more quantitative thinking had to be introduced into perinatal pharmacology than was customary at the time, both in clinical research and teaching. In our unit, for instance, we were ready in 1970 to summarize the state of the art in a supplement issue of the Swedish Medical Journal which was devoted to pediatric pharmacology. Today, 15 years later, the contents seem rather dusty and outdated; much has happened since then. We can now be happy to see several clinical research centers in pediatric pharmacology scattered around the world, some with a more basic profile, some with a more clinical research program. These centers keep relatively good contact with one another. A number of international meetings are arranged and some periodical journals in the area have been launched. Several monographs and reviews are now available.

MAIN ADVANCES

Clinical pharmacology in general has advanced rapidly during the last 20 years. The main achievement has been <u>quantitation</u>, both as regards pharmacokinetics and measurement of the degree of drug effect in the patient. The new possibilities to describe, in detail, the changes with time of drug and drug metabolite concentrations, even when they are extremely low, in blood, urine, cerebrospinal fluid, saliva, etc, were made possible through the impressing advances in analytical technology. The methods today are sensitive, selective, and dependable. In some patient groups, the assay of serum concentrations has been a routine procedure for many years already. Anew disaster of the chloramphenicol type is very unlikely since monitoring of the blood concentration would give early warnings. The very impressing enlargement of our pharmacokinetic knowledge is a good protection for the patient.

This quantitative approach has also revealed that a drug is not simply "a drug". With this I mean two things: first, that the drugs we are using are contained in a pharmaceutical formulation which itself may influence the clinical result, and, secondly, that the drug may be converted to active metabolites which may sometimes contribute to the total effect.

The <u>pharmaceutical formulation</u> may be very important for the clinical result, especially when oral administration is used. But there may be problems also with products given parenterally. An example is the classic report by Leo Stern et al. back in 1971, that the inclusion

of preservative buffers, benzoic acid and sodium benzoate, in the
diazepam injection solution, could displace the protein binding of
bilirubin and thereby induce hyperbilirubinemia.

The second point, the understanding that <u>some drugs may be metabolized to active compounds</u> is a concept with important implications for
fetal and neonatal pharmacology. Drugs are foreign substances to the
body, "xenobiotics". The enzyme systems responsible for biotransformation attack xenobiotics in the same way as they attack physiological
substrates. Thus, the intermediate steps are controlled by enzymes
that recognize certain chemical configurations and the concentration
of each intermediate is controlled both by the enzyme that synthetizes
it and by the enzyme that breaks it down one step further. We have
finally understood that a deficiency of an enzyme activity may either
be a threat to the individual, i.e. if the substrate is toxic and
accumulates, <u>or</u> be protecting the individual if the deficient enzyme
activity would have given rise to a toxic product. No wonder that the
total pharmacological effect may be very different at different
stages in ontogenesis. No wonder that species differences dominate
the scene.

<u>Theophylline</u> may serve as an example. The plasma half-life is about
30 hours in the neonate, which is 5-6 times that of the adult. It was
a small sensation six years ago when French and Canadian groups
reported that neonates were able to produce caffeine when they had
been given theophylline. Such a conversion could not be demonstrated
in adults. Caffeine is a trimethylated xanthine whereas theophylline
is dimethylated. Why should newborn infants but not adults have the
capability to methylate theophylline? Maybe the explanation is that
we have, in all ages, a capacity to methylate but that this capacity
in adults is offset by demethylation and oxidation pathways, which
are not so active in neonates. In other words, when the infant gets
older, often during the first week of age, demethylation taked over
and the result of methylation, i.e. caffeine, is no longer seen. This
maturation of theophylline metabolism may be induced prenatally with
steroids. However, the plasma half-life of theophylline did not
change, as was shown recently by the Westmead Group in Australia.
This shows that plasma level determination is not enough to
characterize drug metabolism. Renal excretion capacity for the
different metabolites must also be taken into consideration.

Another lesson we learned is that the <u>species differences</u> may be so
great that animal studies are of little significance in human
perinatology. The <u>in vitro</u> work on human fetal liver microsomes
during the 1970's showed that the cytochrome P-450 system, as studied
in microsomal fractions, was present at up to 4/5 of the adult levels
and also functionally active in the oxidation of several substrates.
This was unexpected: during more than a decade many papers had been
published that clearly and nicely had demonstrated that laboratory
animals had deficient or absent drug metabolizing activity during the
fetal and neonatal period.

In addition to the species variation it was found that there is also
a considerable <u>inter-individual variation</u> in metabolism of xenobiotics. Both genetical and environmental factors, for instance disease,
contribute to this variation. I think that one of the most important
questions facing developmental pharmacology today is to determine
which these factors are and how they may interact. Better knowledge
about this would give answers to many basic and clinical questions.

We have assumed that the considerable drug oxidative capacity in the human fetus and newborn, relative to laboratory animals, is due to a stronger enzyme induction, but the evidence is not convincing. In fact these enzymes are not easily inducible in the human fetus, at least not with the classical types of inducers which are active in most animals studied. The factors that regulate the time-table for maturation of drug metabolic enzyme function are almost unknown.

Another aspect that has to be considered is the existence of alternative routes for biotransformation. There is considerable flexibility. Glucuronide conjugation is generally poor in the newborn but other pathways, like oxidation and sulfation may compensate. Paracetamol (acetaminophen) has become a popular probe drug since it is conjugated both with glucuronic acid and sulfate. In adults, sulfate conjugates account for 15 to 30 per cent of the dose and 50 to 70 per cent is glucuronic acid conjugates. In newborns, there is the opposite relation. We studied, some years ago, the metabolic fate of phenobarbital in newborn infants with seizures. The cumulative urinary output of phenobarbital and its hydroxylated and conjugated metabolites were measured in 4 infants during 8 days. Two adult volunteers served as controls. It was found that, compared with adults, the infants sere good oxidators but poor conjugators. However, this had more academic than clinical importance since phenobarbital was not critically dependent upon conjugation for its total elimination. Furthermore, these infants had a very good ability to excrete unchanged phenobarbital renally. So, in this case, in the face of the total excretion picture, the low activity in one metabolic channel did not endanger the child.

Most of this type of achievements have been possible only because of progress in analytical technology. The new methodology has also been the basis for the therapeutic drug monitoring (TDM) which is now a safety device in pediatrics, especially in neonatology. A properly run TDM laboratory is a great help both in routine medical care and in evaluation of uncommon events The technical problems (sensitivity, selectivity, reproducibility) have now been largely solved; what bothers me is the increased commercialization in the area with entire analytical equipments for sale, heavily promoted on the market. There is an obvious risk for overuse and misuse of drug analysis: TDM may fall in disrepute if it is used uncritically.

Units for pediatric pharmacology should try to combine more basic pharmacodynamic investigations with studies on practical drug therapy in children. In our case, we tried to analyze autonomic receptor functions in human fetal tissues using the classical isolated organ bath technique, in combination with histochemical mapping with catecholamine fluorescence histochemistry. John Lind was especially interested in our experiments with human ductus arteriosus in vitro. We perfused the isolated ductus and we made spiral strips of it; then we made dose-effect curves of the muscular contraction of such strips after exposure to increasing concentrations of acetylcholine and noradrenaline. The ductus contracted well on both types of stimulation whereas the aorta was not sensitive to noradrenaline. This had its couterpart in the presence of noradrenergic fluorescence in the ductus but not in the aorta, which could be demonstrated in histological sections of the junction between the ductus and the descending aorta. But many questions arose. Is the presence of transmittor a reliable proof of receptor and effector function? For instance, sections of vas deferens from male human fetuses responded persistently with strong contraction upon noradrenaline stimulation and were found to contain abundant fluorescence. Why is this issue so well equipped already during the 15th week of gestation? It has no known function until puberty. The myocardium, on the other hand, which must serve actively already from the start of fetal life, has little fluorescence and low catecholamine content, both in the rat and human, as was shown by Greenberg and Lind back in 1961. The question is: what comes first, nerve endings, transmittor, receptor function, or effector system?

During the first part of the 1960's, the radioreceptor ligand technique which is now so extensively used in most corners the world, was not generally available. The classical technique of studying receptor function, i.e. measuring smooth muscle contraction as a response to graded concentrations of transmittor, seems to be almost forgotten. It is interesting to see that the original enthusiasm for measurement of receptor affinities and receptor population with ligand binding, was somewhat cooled down when warnings for over-interpretation were appearing in the literature. It was said by critics that "half of the definition of a receptor is lost in ligand binding experiments". To characterize binding is not enough, some functional test must also be performed. Thus, formation of c-AMP during beta-adrenergic stimulation has become a common biochemical test for receptor function. More recently, a functional test of histamine 1 receptors has been reported: one measures the in vitro accumulation of ^{3}H inositol-1-phosphate, which is antagonized by H1- but not by H2-histamine antagonists. This type of correlation between binding and biochemical events should be studied during ontogenesis and will no doubt be important for a better understanding of adaptive phenomena during drug therapy like up- and down-regulation of receptors and interaction between pre- and post-synaptic receptor functions. However, this type of in vitro experiments must be interpreted with caution since membrane preparations, like the microsomal P-450 preparations I mentioned earlier consist, after all, of cell fragments and we know that the mode of differential centrifugation, composition of the incubation media, etc, may strongly influence the results.

The growing knowledge in basic developmental pharmacology could be better exploited clinically if more controlled clinical trials were performed in children: first, lack of tradition for this type of study in pediatrics; secondly, paucity of suitable noninvasive techniques; and thirdly, the special ethical restrictions prevailing in pediatric research in general. The lack of tradition and the lack of suitable techniques will gradually disappear. But the ethical restrictions will remain. It is often difficult, or impossible, to apply the common type of protocol for clinical drug testing into pediatrics, especially in neonatology. For instance, there is no such thing in pediatrics as an "informed volunteer". Therefore, it is often a problem to organize an adequate control group, particularly an internal control group with non-treated controls. Externally controlled trials make use of controls from another time period or clinicalsetting, i.e. "historical" controls. Externally controlled studies must avoid many pitfalls but may, critically applied, give important and udeful information. One example in neonatology is the first reports en 1976 on the successful use of indomethacine in persistent ductus arteriosus by Friedman et al. and Heymann et al. They used only historical controls but the principle was rapidly accepted; indomethacine and no other inhibitor of prostaglandin synthesis has become the drug of choice for pharmacologic treatment of PDA.

In some types of drug studies in neonates, it is possible to arrange the protocol in such a way that the burden of risk and discomfort is sufficiently lessened to allow the study. The protocol may be designed so that a trying interference, a venipuncture, a spinal tap, or some clinical measurement, is made only once in each patient. By means of careful planning, a time-concentration or a time-effect curve may still be obtained. For instance, in our studies on the transfer from the mother to the fetus of pethidine (meperidine) and its demethylated metabolite, nor-pethidine, we could reconstruct the kinetics by taking only one umbilical venous and arterial blood sample at delivery and arranging the data along a time axis, i.e. the period between administration and delivery. After about 120 minutes, the concentration of pethidine was higher in the artery than in the vein, indicating the onset of a net back transfer from the fetus to the mother. Such an analysis may help us to interpret the pattern of pethidine and morpethidine concentration in the newborn even if only one single sampling is allowed. In other words, in spite the ethical restrictions, it may be possible to follow the disposition of drug and drug metabolite in a satisfactory way. A similar technique of pooling individual single values was utilized in a further unpublished study where we compared the appearance of pethidine and its metabolite in the CSF of the mother with appearance in the umbilical circulation. It was possible to do this in caesarean section patients who received pethidine as premedication and had spinal anesthesia so we had access to CSF. It was found that the drug appeared earlier in the umbilical vein than in the maternal CSF. This type of "composite" time-curves may be useful for certain kinetic studies in neonatology.

Of course, the gradual progress in non-invasive methodology will also improve the possibilities for pharmacologic evaluations, even if these techniques are primarily designed for diagnostic purposes or directed towards clinical monitoring. Sometimes very simple devices may be sufficient, such as that used by Dr.Wallin in our Department, who time-lapse filmed preterm infants following phenobarbital administration for hyperbilirubin prophylaxis. A very simple equipment was enough. It was found that the sleep pattern, defined as per cent Stage 1 sleep, or non-REM sleep, was correlated to the individual plasma level of phenobarbital at steady state. Except for the capillary sampling, this procedure was entirely non-invasive, and our Etical committee could easily approve the study.

In this rhapsodical account of what has happened in neonatal pharmacology, I have left out much but mentioned some of the things that I know particularly interested John Lind. He helped us all and stimulated us. His sense of humor gave him many friends. Maybe that is part of the explanation for his remarkable ability to raise funds for purposes that he found important. For instance, he found money for a new research building which was ready for use in 1970 and in which, among other activities, our new Department of Clinical Pharmacology was nicely accomodated. He persuaded The Association for The Aid of Crippled Children in New-York to sponsor the first Symposium of Fetal Pharmacology which was held at Skokloster Castle outside Stockholm in 1973. It was still surprising to many that the fetus could have a pharmacology "of its own". We were able to invite many outstanding scientists from all parts of the world. Although did not himself work with drug problems, he was, in my mind, a most important person at the discussions at that Symposium. It is no doubt that John Lind, this remarkable man, also played a role for the development of international developmental pharmacology.

RESUME

Depuis les années 50, de nouvelles possibilités thérapeutiques d'ordre pharmacologique sont apparues en médecine "d'adulte", mais il était nécessaire de les adapter sous forme de données pharmacologiques pédiatriques. Après un rappel historique des cettes évolution, le premier progrès à citer concerne le rôle croissant des méthodes quantitatives en pharmacocinétique et en évaluation des effets thérapeutiques, grâce à des techniques sensibles, sélectives, et fiables. La formulation pharmaceutique peut avoir des conséquences cliniques importantes. D'autre part, certaines substances peuvent être métabolisées en composés actifs, par exemple la théophylline que le nouveau-né est capable de transformer en caféine. Les différences observées selon les espèces, et les variations individuelles sont considérables. Enfin, les voies alternatives de bio-transformation permettent une large flexibilité.

La plupart des nouvelles connaissances ont été acquises grâce aux progrès réalisés dans le domaine des techniques d'analyse, permettant par exemple une surveillance thérapeutique en néonatalogie. L'étude histochimique des catécholamines par fluorescence (par exemple dans la paroi du canal artériel) a montré la présence de tels transmetteurs mais soulève la question de leur rôle fonctionnel? Les méthodes utilisant des marqueurs radioactifs sont maintenant largement répandues.

De plus grands bénéfices seraient tirés de la pharmacologie du développement s'il se faisait davantage d'essais thérapeutiques contrôlés. Les protocoles classiques peuvent être adaptés à la population pédiatrique et même au nouveau-né, aux moindres risques, et en perturbant l'enfant au minimum, en recourant à certaines astuces d'organisation des essais et avec l'aide des nouvelles techniques non-invasives.

Dedication to John Lind
En hommage à John Lind

Space, form and illusion

Jack Metcoff

George Lynn Cross Research Professor, Departments of Pediatrics and Biochemistry and Molecular Biology, University of Oklahoma Health Sciences Center, PO Box 26901, Oklahoma City, OK 73190, USA

Johnny Lind was a cultured man, and culture is no more than a manifestation of the human mind. The process of thinking, of innovating, is a unifying theme which underlies all cultures. The products of culture are secondary, it is the process that is the essential feature. Imagination and creativity are required, both in science and in art, and they share the same process. There are not two cultures, only two groups of individuals: those who innovate and those who do not. Many great scientists were creative artists, for example in United States, Samuel Morse and Robert Fulton were painters. Morse invented the telegraph, but also was one of the greatest American painters of his day. Claude Bernard was a painter of miniatures, perhaps contributing to his skills as an anatomist. Other painters included Humphrey Davis, Pasteur, Helmholtz and Huxley. Galileo, Van t Hoff, Haldane, and Bronowski were poets. Kepler, Planck, Einstein were musicians. The great English phsiologist, A.V.Hill, once said: "I have never known a good scientist who had broad interests.....But I have never known a great one who did not". There are many cross links between scientific and artistic creativity and inventiveness is shared in both fields (1).

How does one get at the process of creativity? You can only infer the process from the products. Can creativity be taught? This is a particularlt relevant question for scientific creativity. Our understanding of the process through which scientific creativity is taught is limited to the product. And that brings us back to Johnny Lind. Johnny successfully accomplished the teaching of creativity in science. That is evidenced by the productive achievement of his students, disciples, and co-workers. The essence of the academic existence is what any of us, as academicians, create. Perhaps our most important creation is not a body of work, but rather our disciples, our students, our pupils. If we are successful with that, we have had an appropriate career. Johnny was spectacular in this regard. His creativity was one of the features which, I think, became evident during the course of this Symposium. The essence of the process for teaching creativity lies in stimulating students to recognize the unknown, to recognize and resolve the problems, to learn how to think for themselves, to invent and not to repeat. In Bronowski's wonderful essay, "Science and Human Values"(2), he states that "science at last respects the scientist more than his theories, for by its nature, it must prize the search above the discovery, and the thinking above the thought". He considered that all science is the search for unity in hidden likenesses, and he claimed that the act of creation in science and in art resides in the discovery of hidden likenesses.

That is the theme underlying my talk: find hidden likenesses. For I shall not attempt to analyze paintings or sculpture, but rather I would like to explore with you some likenesses and try to indicate how some artists discovered new ways of perceiving nature and of expressing their perceptions. Discovery often means simply the uncovering of something which was always there, but was hidden from the eyes by the blinkers of habit. To challenge entrenched dogma in science we must remove these blinkers. That is what I hope we might achieve to-night. I am going to show you something about space. It may not be familiar, for space is dynamic and more than a void that surrounds objects; it limits them and defines form. Form, plus space and light (or color), create an illusion. Form is a symbol; art is an illusion. How we perceive, accept or imagine the illusion determines the extent of esthetic experience.

For those of you who did not know Johnny Lind, this slide (no figure) shows how a contemporary Swedish artist conceived his image. There are those who think that it is a good image, those who object to it. It is very interesting to me because it emphasizes the abstract, intellectual, precise, constrained and controlled emotion characterizing both subject and artist. Johnny was not well when this picture was painted and I think you can almost perceive that. Consequently, the illusion is not the kind one might expect to see in a portrait of an individual who contributed so much, yet it is appropriate because it presents an insight that accents the quality of the individual rather than detracts from it. I thought that bringing Johnny Lind here tonight might be an appropriate illusion to introduce my subject.

My purpose is not to educate, but to stimulate your imagination, to present an opportunity for you to create your own perceptions of space, form and illusion. Some slides may conjure up associations. Some of the paired stimuli will be amusing, some serious, some emotional. Three artists are my nucleus. First, the perception of space as defined by its basic expression, the plane. After 500 years of recognizing space through perspective, and modulated by light, shadow, color, the Cubists reordered space and form into geometrically complex advancing or receding surfaces. Suddenly a new conception emerged which was to change our perception of space and form, and was to stimulate new concepts in architecture, typography, and visual experience (3). The Dutch artist Piet Mondrian created a new kind of space, demarcated by the tension of asymmetrically placed intersecting horizontal and vertical black lines, and emphasized by limited use of the primary colors, red, blue, and yellow, each having a different value to provide a sense of depth. Second, the American artist, Alexandre Calder, who was deeply influenced by Mondrian, retained the primary colors but introduced simple forms -the circle, sphere, and ellipse- taken from the universe, and often squeezed into distorted shapes. And third, the Spaniard Joan Miró, who transformed simple shapes into more complex images, often illusory, suggestive, and amusing, with an extension of paul Klee's idea that a line was "a point with a direction". His images are sharpened by the use of black coupled with the primary colors.

Throughout, the paired slides show paintings or sculpture defining space and form with some paired illusions recorded by the camera. Hidden likenesses are sometimes explicit, sometimes subtle, relating space, form or illusion on one screen to that on the other.

We shall start from the first use of both imagination and perspective. First, a detail of the painting of Joachim's Dream by Giotto in the Capella delle Scrovegni in Padua. Giotto developed the representation of perspective on a flat surface and at the same time created a sense of human emotionality which pervaded the painting unlike anything that had existed before that time, when human forms and conceptions were stylized. Mosso, Giotto's pupil, created an imaginary phenomenon in which he showed St.Sylvester in two different places and positions simultaneously, preparing to raise and raising the dead. The single picture contains not only perspective but an imaginative process involving movement, time, and two separate events, creating the illusion of events in time. That was an enormous creative jump. Perspective in painting was developed, explored and played with, until ultimately it was flaunted as people, objects, even architectural details appeared to project from the flat surface, and ultimately reached the zenith of this expression with Tiepolo, at the end of the Baroque period. When a photograph along the Colorado River and the Grand Canyon is juxtaposed, the shapes, the forms and the colors are identical, and there is a great similarity in the distribution of spatial values in the two scenes. Perspective as an idiom persisted throughout the periods of the various "isms", including Impressionism, as noted in Van Gogh's view of an orchard in Arles. Perspective here is achieved by the classical device of scale, the smaller trees appear further away, providing a sense of depth. In contrast, a single tree in the Ginkagu-Ji, achieves the same sense of perspective: the one tree has red leaves which project it forward and the surroundings make the background recede, but less than the blue of the water, thus depth is perceived. So perspective here is achieved solely by color values, in contrast to the familiar view of the Orchard in Arles. In a very early painting by Mondrian, "The Wood", the sense of perspective also is achieved by the color values with the foreground having the violent reds and yellows and the background containing blacks and thinner lines of color in the trees, thus they are removed in space, and we perceive perspective. The orientation of the trees in Mondrian's picture is not dissimilar from the view of a forest someplace in France, in which the trees proved a linear perspective by their arches. Perspective is related to our common interpretation of visual experience. In the ceiling vaulting of the Gothic church somewhere in France, or the ceiling of Tange's skating rink in Tokyo, the feeling generated by the arches and the lighting are the same, so that we recognize the hidden likeness even though both views represent rather abstract pictures and are separated in time by five centuries. We recognize their similarity because of their familiar perspective. Similarly, with the walls of the Forbidden Palace in China, or the facades of the Grand Arcade in Brussels, the familiar perspective is achieved by the simple linear surfaces receding to a vanishing point.

Then suddenly, at the beginning of the first third of the 20th century, a new concept emerged. The Dutch Painter, Piet Mondrian, created what he called "neoplasticism". What he achieved was to understand that space could be dissociated from perspective; that space could be achieved by the relationship of rectangular planar

surfaces, composed of white or primary colors and demarcated by the
tension between the vertical lines which set off horizontal spaces
and the horizontal lines which set off vertical spaces. And so he
created a series of rectangles, each of which were of different size
and set off by intersecting black bars allocating the space. With
only the use of black lines, white and gray as values, and the
primary colors red, yellow and blue as qualities, his rectangles
create the sense of space, emotion and tension in contiguous small,
variably sized rectangles within a larger rectangle. This early pa
painting has only one colored rectangle: it is red. Although it is
almost the smallest of the rectangles, it projects itself forward so
that you see it immediately and you feel the differentiation of
space (Figure 1, left). He constantly tried to resolve the plasticity
of space by creating new relationships among the rectangles. That
concept of plasticism, neoplasticism, had an enormous impact upon
contemporary architecture, painting and typography formats, all
derived from his conception of space. Mondrian's Composition in Red
and Black is contrasted with the 16th century room in the Kasanji
temple in Kyoto.

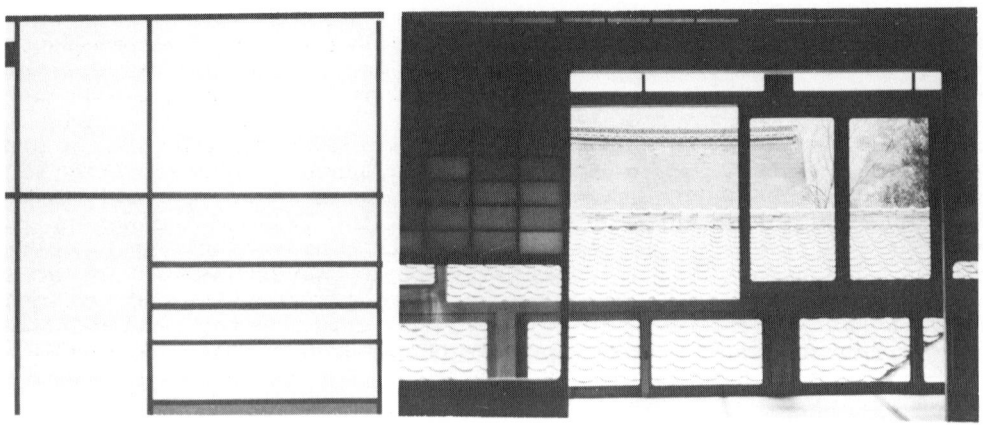

Figure 1.

The Japanese for centuries have related themselves to space by
ordering it with tatami on the floor, and the shoji doors or windows
on the walls of their buildings. Space had a particular, precise
meaning for them. The concept that Mondrian derived hundreds of years
later was really not very much different than that which the Japanese
perceived centuries earlier. Today, wherever you are, you can
perceive the epitome of Mondrian in almost any facade, for example
the characteristic Mondrian, Composition in Red and Yellow and a
facade someplace in Paris. Or another Mondrian, Composition in Red,
Blue and Yellow, and a facade of the Shoin in the Katsura in Kyoto.

The facade bears the same relationship to the plastic flat surfaces, the color highlights, the use of verticals and horizontals to create the tensions and the values perceived later in another culture by Mondrian. In South America and in France, the perception of the facade as a plastic flat space demarcated by horizontal and vertical lines is, I think, everywhere. The last painting of Mondrian's compositions, called Broadway Boogie Woogie, is perhaps his only mature painting which does not have black. He immigrated to New-York in 1930 and died there in 1934. He painted this last picture when he was 61 and called it Broadway Boogie Woogie because he was entranced with New-York. It was said that he loved to dance and that this painting represents a choreographed version of what he considered the excitement of Broadway. The yellow bars with their little blue or red inset rectangles create movement of space and a sense of activity. Although it is obviously a very stationary painting, yet it seems highly mobile and appears to dance with glee. The same sense of movement can be seen in the entrance to the Museum of The Hague. In Brasília, marble cubes, seats, in the cathedral, create another similar kind of space. The juxtaposition of many rectangles having somewhat different color values always have a Mondrian-like quality, whether it is in portraits of children painted by schoolchildren in Osaka, or the postal cards outside of the Blue Mosque in Istanbul.

Alexandre "Sandy" Calder was the fourth generation of artists in his family. His great-great-grandfather was a stonecutter. His great-grandfather was also a stonecutter and a sculptor who worked on the Albert Memorial in London. His grandfather migrated to America in the 1880's, moved to Philadelphia and eventually became a major artist. He constructed the 37-foot statue of William Penn on top of the City Hall in Philadelphia. Sandy's father also was the sculptor of the Swann Fountain in Philadelphia. Sandy's stabile is nearby. It is possible to stand in one spot and see three generations of sculpture by Calders. Calder became intrigued by simple forms as a result largely of a visit he made to Mondrian's studio in Paris in 1930. There, for the first time, he said that he began to understand abstract art. Calder had a great sense of humour and was interested in a wide variety of things. Ultimately his creative interests centered on the Universe, which he took as his "large, live model" (4). He considered that the spheres in the Universe were the essence of form which could be best conveyed with primary colors. He distorted the spheres, squeezing them into somewhat irregular forms.
A poster advertising an annual sculpture event in Basle depicts a Calder mobile. A sculpture in Mexico has some of the same qualities. This Calder "Yellow Disc with Six Red Teeth" (on left, Figure 2) is a tapestry which bears a kind of illusionary similarity to the tops of these parasols seen somewhere in Japan (on right). There are similarities of form, color and emotion between nature and creations of man, a temple lantern in Kyoto related to a barrel cactus in Arizona; or Calder's Red Sun, and the Baroque sun in the garden at Ludwigsburg in Germany. Or his Floating Discs evokes an illusion of light and space like the chandelier in the Kennedy Center. Similarly, Calder's floating swann at the Kroller-Mueller Museum in Holland, and a radar antenna have something of the same form and humorous quality. Similarly, the entrance to the Vasarély's Foundation near Aix, and a view through the moon door of DuFu's cottage in China are related by their black spheres. So is a detail of a wave in the 9 Dragon Scroll from the very remarkable 13th Century Chinese Scroll, and the foot of the Sleeping Buddha in Kyoto, Japan.

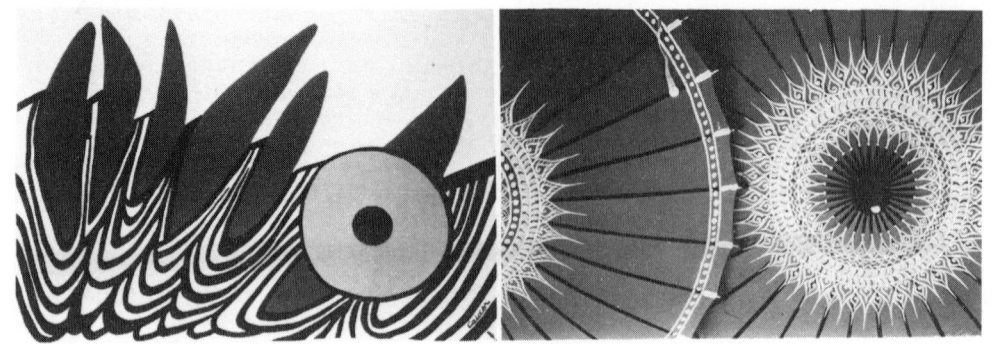

Figure 2.

One of Miró's most significant paintings, "Still Life With an Old Shoe", represents his comment about the destruction of Spain at the end of the Spanish Civil War (5). It suggests to the Spaniard not only the davastation of Spain, but the reduction of life to bread, the crumbling of society, like buildings, and the old shoe perhaps depicts the human condition. Shoes and feet say much about a culture. The symbolism and the illusion they create depend upon our perception and imagination. When you see precisely regimented shoes at a door step, you know immediately you are in Japan, at a holy place, for example the Byodoin. Similarly the bowl and the prayer sheets with clogs identify a Shinto temple, while other details indicate a Zen temple. Feet create an illusion. These boot and shoe forms near the Marais, in Paris, seem to prepare one to be aware of this visitor to the Vasarély Foundation. There are many affinities in portraits; Nefertiti in Berlin and a slum-dweller in Sao Paulo evoke opposite illusions of spiritual repose and spiritual unrest. A painting of a Romanesque Saint in Barcelona and a Klee portrait also evoke similar feelings. A ceramic mural by Miró at Harvard has affinity with the flower "Bird of Paradise" in Honolulu.

The Portrait IV by Miró is both amusing and fear inspiring not unlike the demi-god figures in a Hindu Temple in Bangladesh. Miró's painting, "Figure"(left in Figure 3) does not seem too far removed from these querulous faces seen in a fish-market in Cadiz (right on figure 3) or pre-Columbian figures from Mexico. The "Seated Woman" by Miro relates to a photograph of a 19th Century elegantly dressed mannequin , out of context in a window of a ghost town in Colorado; both comment about social mores through a seated woman. A Nude by Miro and a poster for Escorts in Amsterdam evoke the same illusions. Similarly a torso from the National Portrait Gallery and a painting of the Duchess de Villars and Sister, School of Fontainebleau. "Maternity" by Miró is perhaps less abstract than most of his paintings. The illusion resembles a nursing teen-mother in the Louvre. The artist's perception and comments about maternity differs as illustrated by Picasso and Rubens. Finally, "Red Disc" by Miró

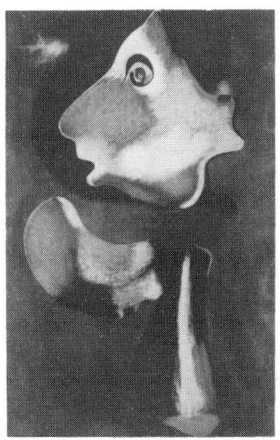 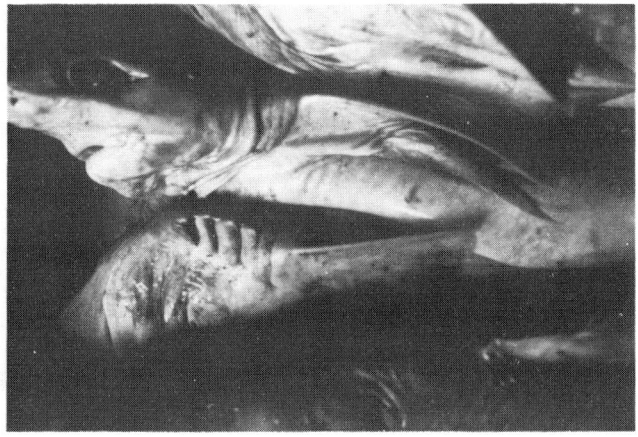

Figure 3.

can be imagined in the sunflowers.

There are also visual illusions that can be seen everywhere if you look. They are paired because of similarities of feeling, not necessarily because of subject matter A rainbow in the "Throat of the Devil" in Iguaçu, Brazil, and another rainbow in Sedona. Communication creates illusions, as in a floating telephone in Colombia (Bogota) and an invitation to 7-up in the desert between Cairo and Alexandria. Or one of the most awful slums in Sao Paulo, dominated by the illusion over it of all the good things in life, while the child in the slum recalls the reality of existence. Other realities: the scribbled "capitalistic church, drug of the people" on a wall in Madrid or the bullets holes in the Berlin Wall, or the cross marking a grave beneath the Berlin Wall and the stones of the Jewish Cemetary in Prague, induce similar devastating illusions.

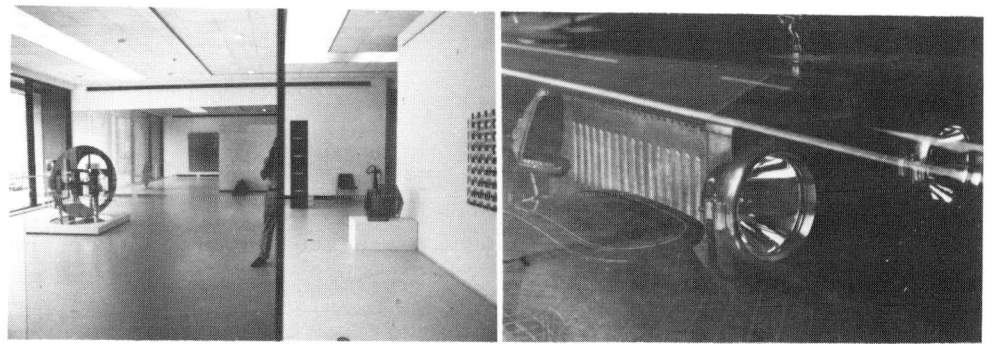

Figure 4.

201

Light also makes curious illusions. Light making unreal shadows on a temple guardian at Nara in Japan or through a window of a Mosque in Pakistan or the glitter of prayer offerings in Chieng Mai, Op art at the Guttai in Tokyo (left on Figure 4), create similar illusions. Finally reflections in glass, like that of an elegant automobile in Spai Spain (right on Figure 4), or the lake and trees reflected in a window of our house are visions leading us to wonder: what is real? What is illusion?

Finally, back to the purpose of this Symposium, to honor Johnny Lind. Is seems fitting to close these comments about Space, Form and Illusion, about Art which meant so much to him, with an illusion of the reality that has passed, the ceramic flowers adorning the graves of the famous deceased at Père Lachaise in Paris, and joy of the present, sign of the new wine, -make the most of life-, the Heurringer.

References.

1. Root-Bernstein R.S. Creative process as a unifying theme of human cultures. Daedalus 1984, 113:197-219.
2. Bronowski J. Science and human values.Harper and Row New-York 1956
3. Gideon S. Space, time and architecture: the growth of a new tradition. Harvard University Press, Cambridge Mass. 1949
4. Lipman J. Calder's universe. Viking Press New-York 1976
5. Soby J.T. Joan Miro. Boubleday New-York 1959.

Participants

René A ARCILLA, M.D., Professor of Pediatrics, Director of Pediatric Cardiology, University of Chicago, Chicago, USA.

Lars O. BOREUS, M.D., Professor and Chairman, Department of Clinical pharmacology, Karolinska Institutet, Stockholm, Suède.

Jacques BOURBON, Chargé de Recherches CNRS, Laboratoire de Physiologie du Développement, Collège de France, Paris, France.

Gerd FAXELIUS, M.D., Department of Pediatrics, Karolinska Sjukhuset, Stockholm, Suède.

Deborah FRIEDMAN, M.D., Assisatant Professor of Pediatrics, Department of Pediatrics, New York University Medical Center, New York, USA.

Bengt FRIIS-HANSEN, M.D., Professor of Pediatrics, Rigshospitalet, Copenhague, Danemark.

Claude GAULTIER, M.D., Professeur Ag. de Physiologie, Hôpital Antoine Béclère, 92 Clamart, France.

Ira H. GESSNER, M.D., Professor and Chief, Pediatric Cardiology, University of Florida, Gainesville, USA.

Petter KARLBERG, M.D., Professor of Pediatrics, Department of Pediatrics, Ostra Sjukhuset, Göteborg, Suède.

Hugo LAGERCRANTZ, M.D., Professor of Pediatrics, Karolinska Institutet, Stockholm, Suède.

Jean LAUGIER, M.D., Professeur de Pédiatrie, Hôpital de Clocheville, 37 Tours, France.

Bo P. LUNDELL, M.D., Ph.D., Karolinska Institutet, Stockholm, Suède.

Giovanna MARCHINI, M.D., Karolinska Institutet, Stockholm, Suède.

Léa MARIN, Chargée de Recherches CNRS, U 29 INSERM, Paris, France.

Jack METCOFF, M.D., Research Professor, Department of Pediatrics, University of Oklahoma, Oklahoma City, USA.

Alexandre MINKOWSKI, M.D., Professeur et Directeur de l'U 29 INSERM, Hôpital Port-Royal, Paris, France.

Pierre MONIN, M.D., Professeur Ag de Pédiatrie, Université de NanceI et INSERM U 272, 54 Nancy, France.

Michèle MONSET-COUCHARD, M.D., Pédiatre Chargée de Recherches INSERM, U29 INSERM, Hôpital Port-Royal, Paris, France.

Guy MORIETTE, M.D., Médicin des Hôpitaux, Service de Médicine Néonatale, INSERM U 29, Hôpital Port-Royal, Paris, France.

William OH, M.D., Professor, Division of Biology and Medicine, Brown University, Providence, USA.

Jean-Pierre RELIE, M.D., Professeur Ag. de Pédiatrie, Service de Médecine Néonatale, INSERM U 29, Hôpital Port-Royal, Paris, France.

Karl G. ROSEN, M.D., Department of Pediatrics, Göteborg Universitet, Göteborg, Suède.

Abraham RUDOLPH, M.D., Professor of Pediatrics, Physiology, and Obstetrics-Gynecology, and Reproductive Sciences, Neider Professor of Pediatric Cardiology, Cardiovascular Research Institute, University of California at San Francisco, San Franciscop, USA.

Bernard SALLE, M.D., Professeur de Pédiatrie, Université Claude Bernard, Hôpital Edouard-Herriot, 69 Lyon, France.

Daniel SIDI, M.D., Chef de Clinique Assistant des Hôpitaux de Paris, Service de Cardiologie Pédiatrique, Hôpital des Enfants-Malades, Paris, France.

Leo STERN, M.D., Professor and Chairman of Pediatrics, Brown University, Rhode Island Hospital, Providence, USA.

Catherine TCHOBROUTSKY, M.D., Maître de Conférences Agrégé, Maternité de Port-Royal, Hôpital Port-Royal, Paris, France.

Paul VERT, M.D., Professeur de Pédiatrie, Université de Nance 1, Chef du Service de Médecine et Réanimation Néonatale, Maternité Régionale Universitaire, et INSERM U 272, 54 Nancy, France.

C. Göran WALLGREN, M.D., Professor of Pediatric Cardiology, Head of the Pediatric Cardiology Department, Karolinska Sjukhuset, Stockholm, Suède.

S. Zoé WALSH, M.D., Research Investigator, Wenner Gren Research Laboratory, Stockholm, Suède.

Hervé WALTI, M.D., Chef de Clinique Assistant des Hôpitaux de Paris, Service de Médecine Néonatale, INSERM U 29, Hôpital Port-Royal, Parris, France.

Joseph WARSHAW, M.D., Professor of Pediatrics, University of Texas Health Sciences Center at Dallas, Dallas, USA.

Alice C. YAO, M.D., Professor of Pediatrics, State University of N.Y. Dowstate Medical Centre, Department of Pediatrics, New York, USA.